SUICIDE-BY-COP
Committing Suicide by Provoking Police to Shoot You

T0358892

by
Mark Lindsay and David Lester

Death, Value and Meaning Series
Series Editor: John D. Morgan

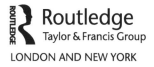

Routledge
Taylor & Francis Group

LONDON AND NEW YORK

First published 2004 by Baywood Publishing Company, Inc.

Published 2018 by Routledge
2 Park Square, Milton Park, Abingdon, Oxon OX14 4RN
52 Vanderbilt Avenue, New York, NY 10017

First issued in paperback 2018

Routledge is an imprint of the Taylor & Francis Group, an informa business

Copyright © 2004 Taylor & Francis

Library of Congress Catalog Number: 2003070869

Library of Congress Cataloging-in-Publication Data

Lindsay, Mark, 1953-
    Suicide by cop : committing suicide by provoking police to shoot you / by Mark Lindsa
and David Lester.
        p. cm. -- (Death, value, and meaning series)
    Includes bibliographical references and index.
    ISBN 0-89503-290-2 (cloth)
        1. Police shootings--United States. 2. Justifiable homicide--United States. 3.
Criminals--Suicidal behavior--United States. I. Lester, David, 1942- II. Title. III. Series.

HV8143.L536 2004
362.28--dc22

                                                                        200307086

ISBN 13: 978-0-415-78534-1 (pbk)
ISBN 13: 978-0-89503-290-4 (hbk)

Table of Contents

SECTION 4
Suicide-by-Cop: A Look at the Issues

The Problem
of Suicide-by-Cop

CHAPTER 1

Introduction

At 10.30 P.M. on November 14, 1997, 19-year-old Moshe Pergament, who was despondent over a $6,000 gambling debt, raced his new Honda Accord along the Long Island Expressway in a rainstorm for 40 minutes, sideswiping other cars. When officer Anthony Sica drew up behind him, with lights flashing, Pergament stopped his car, got out, and drew a gun. Officer Sica shouted for Pergament to drop the gun. Pergament held onto the gun and walked toward Sica. As Pergament drew closer, Sica shot him. The gun turned out to be a plastic replica of a .38 revolver. On the front seat of the Honda was a suicide note addressed "To the officer who shot me." Rebecca Stincelli (undated) has reproduced the note.

> Officer,
> It was a plan. I'm sorry to get you involved. I just needed to die. Please send my letters and break the news slowly to my family and let them know I had to do this. And that I love them very much. I'm sorry for getting you involved. Please remember that this was all my doing. You had no way of knowing.
>
> Moe Pergament.

The medical examiner ruled the death as homicide caused by gunshots, and the police report classified it as a justifiable homicide. These days we call it *suicide-by-cop*.

Sometimes the situation turns into a barricade incident. The offender may be killed by police or he may kill himself. Fuselier, Van Zandt, and Lancely (1991) reported the case of Jimmy Hyams, who on July 18, 1989, had a row with his daughter, Lisa, about her decision to move in with her boyfriend. His wife fled the house with their 7-year-old daughter, and Hyams shot Lisa with a .32 caliber semi-automatic pistol. He closed the door and held off the police for seven hours. He wounded a Suffolk County police officer and eventually killed himself.

The offender does not always get killed. Richard Parent (1998) described a case in August, 1989, in which an officer of the Royal Canadian Mounted Police in a suburb of Vancouver responded to a call about a drunken youth who was threatening his family with a knife. The 15-year-old teenager was hanging out of his broken bedroom window with a bayonet in his bloody hand. The officer entered the house, and the youth rushed the officer waving the bayonet. The officer retreated out to the driveway and back out into the street, pursued by the youth who was uttering threats. Other officers arrived, and the youth was subdued without further incident.

Although these kinds of incidents seem to be occurring with increasing frequency today, they are not a new phenomenon. Nor are they confined to North America. They are an interesting type of suicidal behavior, they often involve criminal behavior such as murder, and they present very difficult law enforcement problems. How should these individuals be handled, and can their lives be spared?

And what is often forgotten, these incidents cause tremendous trauma for the police officers involved. Officer Anthony Sica killed a man holding a toy gun. But he did not know this. Post-traumatic stress disorder is common for the police officers involved in these incidents, and counseling of the officer may be required if he or she is to continue to function effectively as a police officer.

This book will address the issues involved in suicide-by-cop and related phenomena. Chapter 2 will review the research on suicide-by-cop. What do we know about the phenomenon? In the second section (Suicide, Murder, and Cops), Chapters 3 and 4 will review other situations in which individuals commit suicide during confrontations with the police (typically by shooting themselves) and other situations in which police officers kill civilians (civilians who are not necessarily suicidal). These situations have some of the elements found in suicide-by-cop incidents, but differ in important ways.

In the third section (Looking at the Larger Context), we place the phenomenon of suicide-by-cop in a broader context. In Chapter 5, we review phenomena found in other cultures that resemble suicide-by-cop, such as "Crazy-Dog-Wishing-To-Die" among Native Americans in previous centuries. In Chapter 6, we review incidents of individuals running amok in America (or engaging in rampage murders, to use another term), and in Chapter 7, we review the literature on victim-precipitated murder in general. In Chapter 8, we explore the possibility that some murders seek suicide-by-execution, and in Chapter 9 we review the research on murder followed by suicide in general.

Section 4, the final section (A Look at the Issues) reviews some of the issues that suicide-by-cop raises for the criminal justice system. In Chapter 10, we discuss the racial issues involved in suicide-by-cop— does racial bias play a role? Chapter 11 presents some legal issues raised by such incidents. Chapters 12 and 13 discuss law enforcement issues, such as how to conduct hostage negotiations and whether police officers need counseling after being involved in such incidents. Finally, in Chapter 14 we discuss ways in which the incidence of suicide-by-cop might be reduced in our society.

CHAPTER 2
Suicide-By-Cop: What We Know

Suicide-by-cop refers to a situation in which, once police officers arrive on a scene, the individual purposely disobeys orders from the police to lay down his weapon and to surrender. The person then intentionally escalates the potential for the use of force by such acts as threatening the police officers or civilians in the area with a weapon, most commonly a gun. The police officers then are forced to escalate their response, often firing at the individual and killing the person in self-defense or to protect the civilians.

Suicide-by-cop is a lethal method of committing suicide because the would-be suicide knows that police officers are trained in the use of guns (and so in all likelihood will hit their target), are certain to have a gun, and will fire in life-threatening situations.

Richard Jenet and Robert Segal (1985) reported a typical case of suicide-by-cop. The perpetrator called 911 four times after 7 P.M. from a school reporting a burglary in progress. When the police arrived, they saw a man at the window who approached the front door. He opened it and fired one shot at the police officers. The stakeout unit and a police dog unit arrived and began to search the building. The suspect was spotted on the first floor, and he again fired a shot at the police and fled. The police dog detected the man on the second floor, whereupon he said, "I give up." The officers secured the dog but, as the officers approached the man, he crouched down and pointed the gun at them. They shot and killed him. The weapon was a .22 caliber starter pistol and incapable of firing live cartridges.

The man turned out to be a male helper at the school, working split shifts. Seven months earlier, he had been admitted to a local psychiatric hospital after attempting suicide by cutting his wrists, and he was diagnosed as having a depressive neurosis.

Wilson, Davis, Bloom, Batten, and Kamara (1998) described an incident in which a 33-year-old white male was involved in a domestic dispute. When the police arrived, he went into his bedroom and pointed his rifle toward his own chest. He refused to come out, cocked and uncocked the rifle, and begged to be killed. The police tried to get his Rabbi and his psychiatrist to come and talk to him, but both refused. After an hour, police shot tear gas into the bedroom, and a police officer wearing a mask entered the room. The man tore the mask off the officer and shouted "I'll kill you," whereupon the officer shot and killed him.

In another case, a 21-year-old white male entered a police department with a loaded .357 Magnum pistol. He pointed it at the solitary police officer there and occasionally at himself, threatening to kill both of them. He fired two rounds and warned officers outside not to enter. He opened the door and fired at one officer but missed, whereupon two other officers shot and killed him. His blood alcohol level was 0.22%, and his urine indicated amphetamine use. He had been diagnosed as having a major depressive disorder and had previously attempted suicide several times.

Some cases of suicide-by-cop have unique features that may not be relevant to the other cases. For example, Bresler, Scalora, Elbogen, and Moore (2003) reported the case of a middle-aged man who attempted to provoke police officers into killing him (but failed to do so), who had a history of alcohol and substance abuse, and who had suffered severe brain trauma when hit by a truck while walking. After recovering from the coma and surgery, the man suffered from severe depressions and explosive rages. It was during one of his explosive rages that he fired his gun in his house and fled after his wife called the police. The police chased him to a wooded area whereupon he decided to kill himself by having the police shoot him in a gun battle. After an exchange of gunfire, he ran further into the woods and was eventually held at gun point by a farmer's son, allowing the police to arrest him. The incidence of brain damage due to trauma is probably rare in most cases of suicide-by-cop, and so Bresler's case has few implications for the phenomenon in general.

THE INCIDENCE OF SUICIDE-BY-COP

It is difficult to estimate the incidence of suicide-by-cop since there is no official "cause of death" which identifies this type of death. Robert Homant and Daniel Kennedy (2000a) reviewed surveys of incidents of suicide-by-cop and estimated that about 10 percent of incidents of deadly force involve suicide-by-cop. In 1990 in the United States, 289 people were killed by "legal intervention" using a firearm.[1] If the 10 percent estimate for suicide-by-cop is valid, this suggests that about 29 incidents of suicide-by-cop might have occurred that year.[2] In contrast, in 1990 there were 30,484 suicides in the United States (18,185 using firearms) and 25,144 homicides (17,498 using firearms).

THE MOTIVATION FOR
SUICIDE-BY-COP

Clinton Van Zandt (undated) described the profile of the typical suicide-by-cop as follows. He is from the lower social classes and uses aggression as a way of responding to problems. He is seeking death because of depression and guilt, despair, or a desire to punish society for the wrongs it has committed against him. His philosophy of life leads him to view suicide as an unacceptable way of dying, whereas forcing others to kill him is acceptable because this makes him a victim of other people's aggression. Thus, he will provoke the police to kill him, even to the extent of killing innocent people or police officers.

If he has killed a significant other prior to the confrontation with the police, then his death at the hands of the police may serve as a punishment for his crime. This suggests that, although he has apparently rebelled against the norms of society, especially in his violent behavior, he has internalized the values of the society, values which demand that criminal behavior be punished.

Kris Mohandie and Reid Meloy (2000) saw the possible motivations for suicide-by-cop as 1) an attempt to escape the consequences of criminal or shameful behavior, 2) using the confrontation with the police to try to reconcile with a significant other (such as a lover), 3) hoping to avoid the exclusion clauses in insurance policies which operate for the first year or two of taking out the policy,[3] 4) overcoming the moral prohibition against committing suicide, and 5) choosing an efficient method for suicide.

---

[1] There were 316 deaths by legal intervention, 21 of which involved legal executions. Of the rest, 289 involved firearms and six "other" methods.

[2] The number of people killed by legal intervention, excluding executions, is reasonably consistent. In 1991 there were 246 people killed in this way, and 314 in 1992.

[3] David Lester (1988) surveyed life insurance companies and found that the majority have a two-year exclusion clause which permits them to refuse payment if the person commits suicide in that time period. Occasionally companies limit this exclusion period to one year. All companies surveyed, however, refund the premiums paid, sometimes with interest.

They gave an example of this type of suicide-by-cop incident. A civilian police department employee showed up at his estranged wife's house, drunk, in order to try to reconcile with her. She let him in to use the bathroom, but then he refused to leave. She threatened to call the police, but he called them first and hung up on the dispatcher. When the police arrived, he grabbed a replica of a gun, but his son talked him out of confronting them. He was taken away for a psychiatric examination.

Mohandie and Meloy suggested that suicide-by-cop could be viewed as an *expressive* behavior; for example, a means of expressing hopelessness, depression, and desperation, a view of himself as a victim, a need to save face by being forcibly overwhelmed rather than surrendering, a need for power, a way to express feelings of rage and revenge, or a need to draw attention to himself or to his issues. To illustrate this type of suicide-by-cop incident, they presented the case of a man who had been evicted from his house and who had recently lost both parents and a son. He was sporadically unemployed, drank a lot, and was described by associates as "down in the dumps." He confronted the police with a rifle and was shot to death. His manner of death expressed his hopelessness and his view of himself as a victim.

Vernon Geberth (1993) suggested that the two main motives for suicide-by-cop are that having another to kill you lessens 1) the sinfulness of the act and 2) the stigma associated with suicide. Some perpetrators are seeking punishment for their sins, real or imagined, while others do not have the courage to end their lives themselves. Some perpetrators may be seeking publicity in their deaths and so behave in a grandiose manner. Geberth also suggested a role for unconscious motives in that the police officer who kills and thereby punishes the perpetrator may be a surrogate or stand-in for the perpetrator's parents whom the perpetrator hated. The perpetrator ensures his own self-destruction and forces the police officer (who symbolizes a surrogate parent) to kill him, thereby causing the police officer to feel regret and guilt for his actions. Finally, if the perpetrator hates authority or is full of rage, then to die defiantly at the hands of the authority, perhaps killing others in the process, may be satisfying. This motive typically leads to a hostage situation in which the negotiations fail or where the perpetrator is a member of a terrorist or radical political group.

It should be remembered that not all suicide-by-cop incidents are the same. In particular, some involve simple confrontations between the perpetrator and the police while others involve hostages and barricade situations. The former last a few minutes, the latter can last for several hours.

STUDIES OF SAMPLES OF
SUICIDE-BY-COP

Richard Parent (1998a) found in British Columbia (Canada) that, from 1980 to 1995, there were 58 incidents in which municipal police officers or the Royal Canadian Mounted Police were confronted with potentially lethal threats. In 27 of these incidents (47%), the police killed the perpetrators; in the remaining cases, no one was killed. In 28 of the incidents (48%), Parent judged the situation to be one of suicide-by-cop; in the incidents in which the perpetrator was killed by police officers, 54 percent were judged to be suicide-by-cop. In these cases, the perpetrator provoked the officers, often with a lethal weapon, and indicated suicidal intent. In many of the cases, the perpetrator was later found to have a documented history of mental illness or suicidal tendencies and was found to be drunk at the time of the incident (or under the effects of drugs).

Vivian Lord (2000) noted that some of the perpetrators may make detailed plans for the confrontation with the police, while others may be more impulsive, reacting only after the police arrive. Lord identified 64 cases of potential suicide-by-cop incidents from 32 law enforcement agencies in North Carolina between 1992 and 1994. Sixteen of the perpetrators were killed by police officers, five killed themselves, and 43 survived. Her cases were primarily white (75%), male (95%), between the ages of 25 and 40 (84%), and in possession of a gun (73%). A quarter were unemployed, and two-thirds had lived in the area for a long time. They lived with partners, parents, or extended families, and were not transient, lonely people. One-quarter of the incidents lasted more than five hours, and the perpetrator was less likely to be killed the longer the confrontation. Forty-three percent of the perpetrators who were killed were killed in the first hour. The most common motive for suicide-by-cop was the break-up of a relationship or other family problems. One-third had talked of suicide prior to the confrontation. Only a quarter were drug or alcohol abusers, but two-thirds were intoxicated with drugs or alcohol during the confrontation with police.

Lord found fewer confrontations during the winter and fewer in the morning. In almost half of the confrontations, other people or the media were present, often contributing to the escalation of the confrontation. In one case, a domestic dispute between a man and a woman, both high on cocaine and alcohol, there were over a hundred bystanders present who encouraged the perpetrator to kill himself or assault the police. He rushed at the police brandishing a knife and was shot and killed. The most common situation leading to suicide-by-cop was suicide intervention, followed by domestic violence intervention.

Some 54 percent of the perpetrators were judged to be mentally ill, and the most common diagnoses were schizophrenia and bipolar affective disorder (more commonly known as manic-depressive illness). More than half of the perpetrators were substance abusers and three-quarters used alcohol and/or drugs during the incident. Only 8 percent were social isolates, and three-quarters had lived in the region for more than a year. Some 62 percent were unemployed, and 89 percent had recently experienced stressful life events, the most common of which was termination of a relationship (30%), followed by family problems (19%) and stress from mental illness (16%). A quarter had shown previous suicidal behavior, and 58 percent made presuicidal communications to significant others (relatives and friends). Half had prior criminal records, most commonly for domestic violence.

As mentioned previously, 16 of the 64 cases resulted in the perpetrator's death, 18 were committed to mental hospitals, 15 were arrested for assault (on police officers or family members), and 9 were injured by the police officers.

Lord grouped together the perpetrators who died, who were injured, and who committed suicide ("successful") and compared them with those who surrendered or who were apprehended ("unsuccessful"). The "successful" perpetrators more often abused hard drugs and less often abused alcohol, were more often non-residents of the region, and were more often involved in criminal activity at the time of the incident. The "successful" perpetrators less often used alcohol during the incident and more often had a history of mental institution commitments,[4] previous suicide attempts, and financial problems, possessed a gun, and mentioned homicide during the incident.

Lord felt that the suicide-by-cop perpetrators resembled ordinary completed suicides (those who die as a result of their own suicidal actions) in some ways, including age and sex, mental illness, alcohol and drug use, stressful life events, unemployment, and anger. However, they differed from ordinary completed suicides in rarely having made prior suicide attempts, not being socially isolated or divorced/separated, and not having physical illnesses. The impulsivity in some cases and the lack of certainty of dying also led Lord to see these actions as similar in some ways to attempted suicides (those who survive their own suicidal actions).

---

[4] Surprisingly, more of the successful perpetrators were also judged to have no mental illness.

Lord noted three types of suicide-by-cop perpetrators: those involved in chronic domestic disputes, those mentally ill, and those trying to avoid arrest for outstanding criminal warrants. The suicide-by-cop situations resulted in the death of the perpetrator more often if they had outstanding criminal warrants, and Lord thought that these men might be motivated by a desire to avoid apprehension and prison. The domestic disputes and mentally ill perpetrators may have been trying to gain some control over their lives.

Range Hutson and his colleagues (1998) reviewed all officer-involved shootings in the Los Angeles County Sheriff's Department from 1987 to 1997 and found 46 incidents of suicide-by-cop. These incidents accounted for 46 percent of all office-involved shootings and 13 percent of officer-involved justifiable homicides. Thirty-nine percent of the incidents involved domestic violence incidents. Ninety-eight percent of the perpetrators were male, primarily white or Latino, and 48 percent of them possessed firearms, with 17 percent possessing replicas of firearms. Seventy percent of the shootings occurred within 30 minutes of the police arriving, and the average time was 15 minutes. Fifty-four percent of the perpetrators died and were classified by the medical examiner as homicides. Hutson noted that suicide-by-cop incidents result in an underestimate of the suicide rate in a community since they are not labeled as suicides in official records.

Sixty-five percent of the perpetrators communicated their suicidal intent to others, 43 percent exhibited signs of suicidal behavior, and 22 percent left written communications (such as suicide notes). Fifty-nine percent asked the police officers to kill them, and 15 percent continued to point their firearm at the police after being warned they would be shot. Sixteen percent lunged at the police with a knife.

Half of the incidents occurred at the person's home, 22 percent at someone else's home, and 28 percent at-large in the community. In 96 percent of the cases, the police had time to try to dissuade the person to lay down their weapon, but to no avail. In a quarter of the cases, the police used less lethal weapons first, such as rubber bullets, bean bag guns, pepper spray, police dogs, tear gas, and Tasers.

At least 70 percent of the perpetrators had prior arrests or convictions, 65 percent were alcohol or drug abusers, 63 percent had a psychiatric history, and 39 percent had been involved in domestic violence incidents.

Kennedy, Homant, and Hupp (1998) searched newspapers for the period 1980 to 1995 and found 240 incidents of police shootings. The civilians involved were typically men between the ages of 16 and 35. Only 5 percent were homeless or mentally ill. Most of the police officers involved were in uniform, and the most common circumstances were domestic disturbances, general disturbances, and "person with a weapon" calls. The most common precipitant was pointing or firing a gun at a police officer. Of these, 160 incidents had too little information to make a judgment. Of the rest, 37 were probably or possible suicide-by-cop incidents while 43 were not suicides or unlikely to be suicides. The suicide-by-cop incidents tended more often to be fatal and to involve the perpetrator pointing or firing a gun or reaching for a weapon.

Edward Wilson and his colleagues (1998) described 15 incidents of suicide-by-cop occurring in Florida and Oregon. All the perpetrators were men, and most were white. All resisted arrest and verbally threatened homicide during the incidents. Eleven had a handgun, three had knives, and one an iron bar. Sixty percent actually used the weapon during the incident. Forty percent were intoxicated with alcohol. Seven of the 15 perpetrators had made attempts at suicide in the past, and 60 percent had clear psychiatric disorders.

Rebecca Stincelli (undated) reported a study by Karl Harris in 1988 that reported that most suicide-by-cop incidents occur on Wednesday and Thursday nights between the hours of 8 P.M. and 10 P.M. Most perpetrators were under the influence of drugs or alcohol, aged 21 to 35, and displayed handguns or knives.

A SUMMARY

Homant, Kennedy, Hupp, and Real (2000) have conveniently summarized these studies for us. They collected together 123 suicide-by-cop incidents from several sources (including some of those reviewed above) and coded the information from each case. The perpetrators possessed firearms in 50 percent of the incidents, followed by a knife in 20 percent. In 22 percent of the incidents, it turned out that the police were not in any real danger—in 9 percent of these incidents the perpetrator had a firearm that was not loaded and in 12 percent the perpetrator used a toy firearm or an object that resembled a firearm.

The police shot and killed the perpetrator in 72 percent of the incidents, in 6 percent the perpetrator committed suicide, in 8 percent the perpetrator was wounded by the police and survived, in 9 percent the perpetrator was overcome, and in 4 percent the perpetrator surrendered or the police left without incident.

Eighty-nine percent of the perpetrators were male, and their ages ranged from 15 to 80, with a mean age of 32. Personal psychopathology or stress was reported for 76 percent of the perpetrators, most commonly family/domestic problems (33%) and drug/alcohol problems (33%). Some 22 percent had previously documented mental illness and 20 percent a criminal history. Fifteen percent had made previous suicide attempts. Twenty-seven percent had clear evidence that the perpetrator was planning suicide, and in 24 percent of the cases this was probable. A fatal outcome was much more likely when others were present at the scene of the incident.

A TYPOLOGY OF
SUICIDE-BY-COP INCIDENTS

Robert Homant and Daniel Kennedy (2000a) took a sample of 145 cases of suicide-by-cop and 29 incidents that did not quite meet the criteria for such incidents. The 29 incidents that did not meet the criteria were standoff or barricade situations, desperate escapes, interrupted suicides, and mistakes in which the police or the perpetrator reacted too quickly (such as in response to a sudden movement).

Homant and Kennedy found four categories of these incidents, each with several subtypes:

1) Direct confrontation
   i) Kamikaze attacks. In these, the perpetrator plans an attack on the police in order to be killed by them, and he makes a direct attack on the police.
   ii) Controlled attacks. Here the perpetrator confronts the police, perhaps approaching them while holding a gun, and demands that they kill him.
   iii) Manipulated confrontations. The perpetrator causes the police to investigate a situation, for example, by calling them to report a crime or a suicide attempt.
   iv) Dangerous confrontations. These incidents are similar to (iii) but the perpetrator actually commits a crime or poses a danger to hostages.

2) Disturbed intervention
   i) Suicide intervention in which the officers are called to prevent an individual from committing suicide.
   ii) Disturbed domestic conflicts in which the police officers respond to a domestic dispute which escalates into a suicide-by-cop incident.
   iii) Disturbed person incidents involve disturbed individuals acting strangely and dangerously. When the police are called, the incident escalates into a suicide-by-cop incident.

3) Criminal intervention

i) Major crime (such as burglary). The police arrive on the scene and prevent the perpetrator's escape. The subject appears to prefer death to arrest and acts so as to force the police to kill him.

ii) Minor crime (such as a traffic stop). Here the perpetrator appears to resist the police intervention, and the resistance escalates.

Homant and Kennedy (2000b) found that the perpetrators were youngest in the criminal intervention incidents (mean age 26) and oldest in the disturbed interventions (mean age 36).[5] But the ages varied also by subtype. The danger to police and others was less in the direct confrontations, while the danger to the perpetrator did not vary with the type of incident. The distribution of female perpetrators among the three major types was similar to that for men.

It is important with typologies to explore the reliability of the classification. Using two people to rate the cases, Homant and Kennedy (2000a) found that there was 96.5 percent agreement on which incidents were not suicide-by-cop, 78 percent agreement for sorting into the three major types of situations, and 60 percent agreement for sorting into the nine subtypes of situations.

A reliable typology is useful because the typology may lead to predictions of the outcome for the police and for the perpetrator and, with increasing experience with the use of the typology, it may be possible to vary the approach taken by the responding law enforcement officers depending upon the type of situation.

HOW ARE THESE DEATHS CLASSIFIED?

Range Hutson (1998) and his colleagues argued that the term suicide-by-cop is a poor term. These deaths are really assisted-suicides and so should be called law enforcement-forced-assisted suicides because they are cases of assisted-suicide in which the police officer is forced to participate. However, Edward Wilson and his colleagues (1998) noted that there is no uniformity in how these deaths are certified by coroners and medical examiners. Some coroners argue that such deaths should be certified as homicides while others argue that they should be certified as suicides.

Randy Hanzlick and Julia Goodin (1997) gave a typical case of suicide-by-cop to 198 medical examiners and coroners and asked them how they would certify it. Eighty-two percent classified it as a homicide,

---

[5] The mean age in the direct confrontations was 31.

11 percent as a suicide, 4.6 percent as undetermined, and 1.5 percent as an accident. The majority would classify it as a homicide even if the suicidal intent of the perpetrator was obvious. However, the National Center for Health Statistics classifies the cause of such deaths as "legal intervention."

CLUES TO POTENTIAL SUICIDE-BY-COP SITUATIONS

How can police officers decide whether an incident is a suicide-by-cop incident? Clinton Van Zandt (undated) provided a list of features of police-citizen confrontations which suggests that they may be suicide-by-cop situations.

1. the person in a hostage/barricade situation refuses to negotiate with the police
2. he has killed a significant other, especially a child or mother
3. he demands that the police kill him
4. he sets a deadline for the police to kill him
5. he has recently learned that he has a life-threatening illness or disease
6. he indicates that he has an elaborate plan involving prior thought and preparation for his death
7. he says that he will surrender in person only to the officer in charge
8. he indicates that he wants to "go out in a big way"
9. he presents no demand that includes his escape or freedom
10. he is from the lower social classes
11. he provides the authorities with a "verbal will"
12. he appears to be looking for a macho or manly way to die
13. he has recently given away money or personal possessions
14. he has a criminal record that includes assaults and violent behavior
15. he has recently experienced two or more traumatic events in his life involving his family or himself
16. he expresses feelings of hopelessness and helplessness.

Kris Mohandie and Reid Meloy (2000) have also listed a set of clues which indicate that an incident may be suicide-by-cop.

Verbal clues include:

1. demands that the authorities kill him/her
2. setting a deadline for them to kill him/her

3. threatening to kill or harm others
4. wanting to go out in a blaze of glory or indicating that he/she will not be taken alive
5. giving a verbal will
6. telling hostages or others that he/she wants to die
7. looking for a macho way out
8. offering to surrender to the person in charge
9. indicating elaborate plans for his/her own death
10. expressing feelings of depression and hopelessness
11. emphasizing that jail is not an option
12. making Biblical references, especially to the Book of Revelations and resurrection.

Behavioral clues include:

1. demonstrating a weapon
2. pointing the weapon at the police
3. clearing an opening in the barricade in order to shoot
4. shooting at police
5. reaching for a weapon with police present
6. attaching the weapon to his/her body
7. counting down to kill hostages or others
8. assaulting or harming hostages
9. forcing a confrontation with police
10. advancing on police when told to stop
11. calling police himself to report a crime in progress
12. continues acts of aggression after being wounded
13. self-mutilation with police present
14. pointing weapon at self
15. refusing to negotiate
16. making no demands to escape
17. making no demands at all
18. getting intoxicated in order to increase his/her courage.

These sets of clues need to be explored in future research for their reliability and validity. Do they predict suicide-by-cop incidents accurately, and are all of the clues equally relevant for this prediction?

SECTION 2

Suicide, Murder, and Cops

CHAPTER 3

Suicide during Confrontations with Police

Suicide of suspects and offenders during confrontations with police is quite common. Since a suspicious public sometimes accuses the police of covering up the murder of suspects by law enforcement officers, investigation of these deaths should be conducted carefully by law enforcement agencies and by medical examiners so that we can be confident that the deaths are suicides.

Harruff, Llewellyn, Clark, Hawley, and Pless (1994) examined 14 cases of suspects committing suicide with a firearm during confrontations with police between 1984 and 1992 in Marion County, Indiana, which includes Indianapolis. All of the subjects were men, and 72 percent were 20 to 39 years of age. Seventy-one percent were white, and 78 percent shot themselves in the head with a handgun, most commonly in the right temple. Fifty-seven percent occurred after a marital or relationship dispute, and 29 percent of the subjects were wanted for a crime. Of the 12 subjects who were tested for alcohol, three had high concentrations of alcohol in their blood.

These 14 firearm suicides accounted for 2 percent of all firearm suicides in the area in that period and 54 percent of all police-involved fatal shootings.

In one of the cases, a 23-year-old black male was holding his 15-year-old girl-friend hostage in an apartment. The police fired tear gas into the apartment but, when they entered, they found both dead from gunshots. In another, a 17-year-old white male was wanted for burglary of an auto-parts store. The police pursued him to an interstate highway rest area where he held them off for two and a half hours. He then shot himself with a .22 caliber handgun.

Three of the subjects were contemplating suicide before the incident occurred, seven were distraught but not suicidal, and four did not appear to have been suicidal until the confrontation with the police.

Dwayne Fuselier and his colleagues (1991) at the FBI presented several cases of hostage/barricade incidents in which the perpetrator committed suicide, and they also presented a profile of the typical perpetrator.

In one case, on Tuesday, August 1, 1989, Manny Cabano walked into the Tarrant County Courthouse, pointed a .357 magnum revolver at Juanita Hermosillo, with whom he had been living for a year, and ordered everyone else out of the building. After a seven-hour stand-off, he killed Juanita and then committed suicide.

Fuselier noted the following components of the profile:

1. The subject has experienced several stressors. In Cabano's case, he was a bail bondsman and several of his clients had skipped bail, thereby leaving him with financial losses. He was on the verge of bankruptcy, and he was being evicted from his home for failing to pay the mortgage. Juanita, who had five children from a previous marriage, had filed charges against him for child sexual abuse and had obtained a court order preventing Cabano from entering her residence.

2. The subject's cultural background involves male dominance. Cabano felt that the charges of child sexual abuse had caused him to lose face. He felt that he could no longer hold his head up in the community, for people would always ridicule him for molesting a child even if he were found innocent. His Hispanic heritage stressed the importance of a man having the respect of others.

3. The subject has a history of similar incidents. Juanita had filed charges of sexual abuse against Cabano in 1988 but then withdrew them. After the relationship soured and Cabano had moved out, Juanita filed the charges again. A year earlier, Cabano had barricaded himself with Juanita and one child in a bedroom and threatened to kill them and himself. One of his ex-wife's co-workers persuaded him to end the siege before the police were called.

4. The subject lacks family and social support systems. Fuselier did not give any details on Cabano relevant to this point.

5. The subject has problematic behavior patterns.

i. The subject forces the confrontation with the police. After ordering everyone from the building, Cabano waited for the police whom he knew would be called.

ii. The subject threatens or injures the victim. In negotiations with the police, Cabano wanted only two bottles of soft drinks and to make a statement to the media, but he was unwilling to release Juanita in return. Eventually he killed her.

    iii. The subject indicates that he intends to commit suicide. Just before entering the courthouse, Cabano gave away his car and a large amount of money. During the incident, he called his ex-wife (a call of which the police negotiators were unaware) and told her to take some items from his safe and destroy them because he would no longer need them.

Fuselier distinguished between hostage situations and pseudo-hostage situations. In hostage situations, a person is held and threatened by the perpetrator in order to obtain the fulfilment of some demand. In pseudo-hostage situations, the victim is threatened or harmed, but there are no demands made to a third party. In the Cabano incident, Cabano wanted nothing in exchange for Juanita's release. Juanita was *not* a bargaining chip.

When should police officers make a tactical intervention in these situations? Fuselier suggested three criteria.

1. Is the action necessary? Is an action being recommended simply in order "to do something"? Is there any reason to engage in the action now rather than later?

2. Is the action risk-effective? Will the action increase the risk to the hostage? Can the chances of saving the hostage safely be increased by one particular tactical action rather than by an alternative?

3. Is the action professionally acceptable? Police departments should set up guidelines for legally acceptable tactical actions. Ethical and moral guidelines are more difficult to prescribe, but they are often relevant. Fuselier gave an example of a father whose 16-month-old boy had been on life support for eight months with little chance of ever recovering consciousness. He went to the hospital room with a handgun, ordered the staff out, and disconnected the life-maintaining equipment from his son. He then cradled the child in his arms, crying, until the child died. The father could have been shot and the child reconnected to the equipment, but such an action would be viewed as unethical to some commentators.

CHAPTER 4

Justifiable Homicide by Police

Clinton Van Zandt (undated) noted that FBI statistics indicate that between 1981 and 1990, a 10-year period, 3.7 million assaults occurred on police officers, and some 617 thousand individuals were identified in these assaults. During the same period, 841 police officers were killed by 1,179 identifiable assailants. Of these cop killers, 798 had prior arrest records, 976 were subsequently charged, 152 were justifiably killed by police, and 45 killed themselves. Thus, 197 of the 1,179 assailants (152 + 45 = 17%) may have had suicidal desires which may have motivated in part their confrontation incident with the police.

The use of deadly force by police officers has been the subject of much concern to policy makers and to the public. When is it appropriate and when is it not? William Geller and Michael Scott (1992) noted four types of factors which influence the decision of police officers to use deadly force.

1. The characteristics of the participants, including characteristics of the suspect (such as his age, race and demeanor) and characteristics of the police officer (such as whether he had a partner present and whether he was a rookie).

2. The circumstances, such as the time of day, a public versus a private setting, the lighting and weather, whether cover was available for the suspect and officer, and the distance between them.

3. The actions of the suspect, including the suspect being uncooperative, unresponsive, or mentally deranged, whether he had a weapon and pointed it toward the officer, whether he was committing a crime, and if there was more than one suspect.

4. The decisions made by the police officer, such as his perception that his own or another's life was in danger.

In many circumstances, the decision to employ deadly force, even to the point of killing the suspect, is judged, after investigation, to have been justified.

A justifiable homicide is an intentional killing either commanded or authorized by the law. One class of justifiable homicides is those in which a police officer kills a suspect or offender.

Gerald Robin (1963) studied all offenders killed by police officers in Philadelphia in the 1950s, a total of 32 people killed by 42 police officers. All died as a result of gunshot wounds, and 11 of the police officers also sustained injuries (ranging from bites to stab wounds). Most of the incidents took place on the street between 9 P.M. and 3 A.M.

Twenty-four of the offenders had committed felonies, such as burglary, robbery, and aggravated assault. When the police tried to arrest the suspects, seven fled, six resisted, and 19 assaulted the officers. In 28 cases, the officer warned the suspect verbally or by firing into the air. The suspects as a group had been charged on an average of almost five times, including just over two felony charges. Two-thirds had served time.

Most of the victims were black (88% versus 31% of all offenders and a city population that was 22% black). The death rates from this type of homicide were 0.55 per 100,000 per year for blacks and 0.03 for whites. The average age of the offenders was 28, with a range of 15 to 60. Only two were juveniles. The majority were unskilled workers,

Robin felt that almost all of the cases were justified, and that the police officers' use of force was authorized by regulations and used as a last resort.

Arthur Kobler (1975) used a nationwide newspaper clipping service and identified 911 incidents of civilians killed by police officers in the 1960s. The description of the incidents resembled that given by Robin, but Kobler was less willing to view all of the acts as justified. For example, he noted that in one-third of the cases, the only witnesses were police officers, and he doubted that their evidence was trustworthy. He judged that about 16 percent of the killings were unjustified, and in four-fifths of these cases the police officer admitted error. Similarly, Richard Harding and Richard Fahey (1973) found that the police in Chicago judged only 1 percent of the killings there to be unjustified, whereas the researchers reckoned that 15 percent were probably unjustified. A typical case of unjustifiable homicide is:

On March 3, 1971, Attorney General Mitchell announced the indictment of four California policemen for violation of civil rights of two Mexican nationals, cousins, aged 22 and 23. On July 16, 1970, the police, seeking a murder suspect, had "mistakenly" stormed an apartment and killed two innocent and unarmed men, neither the suspect nor any arms being found in the apartment. (Kobler, 1975, p. 180)

DISCUSSION

This book is concerned with suicide-by-cop situations, in which an individual acts in such a way as to force police officers to shoot and kill him. It is critical, therefore, that such cases be distinguished from cases in which the suspect shoots himself during confrontations with the police (as described in Chapter 3) and situations in which police officers unjustifiably use deadly force and kill suspects (as described in the present chapter). Friends and relatives of deceased suspects often accuse the police officers involved in incidents of suicide-by-cop and where suspects commit suicide of using unjustified deadly force. If we study and come to understand suicide-by-cop incidents better, we may be able to reassure community residents that their police forces can be trusted to use deadly force circumspectly and justifiably.

SECTION 3

Looking at
the Larger Context

CHAPTER 5

Similar Behavior in Other Cultures

Many other cultures have behaviors (or syndromes) in which people become violent toward others and are themselves killed. One of the common terms in our language for this is "berserk." John MacDonald (1961) suggested that this term comes from Norse (Scandinavian) mythology in which Starkadder, who had eight hands, and Alfhilde had a grandson named Berserk, who was named for the furious way he went into battle without wearing armor, increasing the chances therefore of being killed. His name, Berserk, was derived from the bearskin he wore as a shirt (ber sark) and was applied to groups of marauders found in the Viking community from 870 A.D. to 1030 A.D., after which they were banned by law.

These men who went berserk were characterized by a wild fury which increased their strength and made them insensitive to pain. They behaved like wild animals and killed everyone they met, friend or foe. Afterwards, they would be exhausted and physically feeble for days. Howard Fabing (1956) suggested that this state was brought on by eating toxic mushrooms which brought on temporary psychoses, but he notes that others have suggested that it was simply an ecstatic fury appearing in a group of aggressive psychopaths.

CRAZY-DOG-WISHING-TO-DIE

Karin Andriolo (1998) has described a number of cultures in which people commit suicide by getting others to kill them. For example, among the Plains Indians, such as the Crow, a man who was tired of living would tell his kin that he wanted to seek death in battle. His relatives would try to dissuade him but, if he persisted, would go along with his choice. The man was now accorded special status. He wore special clothes, used a special rattle, and danced and sang special songs.

In these he would talk "crosswise," that is, expressing the opposite of his real intentions and doing the opposite of what he was told. He was allowed to eat whatever he wished and to have sex with whomever he desired. His death in battle would then become a glorious memory for the tribe to recall and re-tell. If he failed to be killed, he was released from his vow and accorded high prestige. If he changed his mind or fled, he was ridiculed and scorned.

Andriolo noted that this form of suicide was not open to women. The women in these societies who killed themselves did so in conventional ways and were stigmatized because ordinary suicide was frowned upon. It appears, therefore, that in these societies men were considered of superior worth than women, and their interests were favored by the cultural norms.

This method of committing suicide has been called *indirect* suicide, *vicarious* suicide, or *masked* suicide. Masked suicide is a public performance and, therefore, a public property. The suicide conforms to the cultural norms and values and thus confirms them. The suicidal person of this type also does not act impulsively, but rather seeks a cause, and the scenario offers solemnity, symbolism, and purpose. The ritual induces control and calmness in the suicide. Robert Lowie (1913) has provided an example.

> Hunts-to-die knew of another Crazy Dog, who lived in his grandfather's time. He was the handsomest Indian ever seen, and was called Good-crazy-dog; his real name was He-strikes-the-enemy-with-his-brother. At one time the Sioux attacked a Crow band, killing all, including some of Good-crazy-dog's relatives. Good-crazy-dog said, "I am going to die, I will be a Crazy Dog." He bought red flannel for the sashes, making one for each side. He made a rattle out of a buffalo paunch, and tied eagle feathers to one end of it; inside he put beads and little stones. He wore a fine war-bonnet on his head and tied skunk skin ornaments to his moccasins. His necklace was of bapà'ce shells, and his earrings of sea-shells. In the back he wore a switch and in front little braids of hair. He rode a fine spotted horse with docked tail; for its trappings he sewed together red and green flannel. When he rode through the camp. he began to sing and the old women cheered him. He was killed in battle. (Lowie, 1913, p. 194)

JURAMENTADO

Andriolo noted also that in Muslim societies, which typically disapprove of suicide in general, dying in the context of a *jihad*, a religious obligation, is considered a glorious death which enables the deceased to enter heaven immediately. In *juramentado*, a man who wished to die would go to a place where there were many Christians and kill as many as possible before being killed.

Andriolo gave examples from the Muslims of the Philippines. Today, these deaths are seen in the suicide bombers in Middle Eastern countries, who tie bombs to themselves or drive cars loaded with bombs to a crowded street and die in the explosion.

This pattern is also found in the Jivaro of Peru and the Yanomano of Venezuela.

> . . . when a [Jivaro] man "no longer wants to live," he does not commit suicide in the ordinary sense, but rather suddenly starts leading assassination raids against the men who are his enemies, insisting on taking the principal risks, such as being the first to charge into the enemy's house. Sooner or later, of course, he will himself be killed, which apparently surprises no one. . . . (Michael Harner, 1972, p. 181)

RUNNING AMOK

Running amok is no mere figure of speech, but a real homicidal syndrome. Dr. B. G. Burton-Bradley (1968) has provided an eyewitness account of such a case.

The subject approached some of his relatives and the witness at dusk one evening while they were sitting outside a house. The subject had a spear, which he threw at one of the relatives, who was hit in the side. The victim was carried inside the house by some of the others. While this was being done, the subject threw another spear which hit another relative, who removed it herself. All ran away, defending themselves in the process. The eyewitness reported that the subject said. "Where are you all? I am coming after you." The witness hid until daybreak. He then found two bodies, one inside the house and one outside. With five other villagers, he searched for the subject and found him in the bush wounded in the chest, with five spears stuck in the ground beside him. He was then overpowered by the villagers. In addition to having attacked and killed people, he had damaged and destroyed yams in the yam house.

When arrested, the subject said that he had been in the bush for two days without food prior to the offense. He claimed to have amnesia for his acts but admitted that it was said that he had killed a man and a woman and speared three others. However, he later admitted that at the time of the offense he was aware that his actions were wrong in the eyes of both his own people and the administration, and that they might lead to his death. He was evaluated at a psychiatric hospital, but no mental disorder was noted.

Amok is a behavior characterized by previous brooding, homicidal outbursts, persistence in reckless homicide without apparent motive, and a claim of amnesia. It is most commonly known as a behavior of the Malays in Malaysia. Various authors have seen its cause in malaria, pneumonia, syphilis infections which have spread to the brain, hashish, heat stroke, paranoid states, and mania. However, Dr. P. Van Wulfften-Palthe (1936) suggested that running amok is a standardized form of obtaining emotional release. The community recognizes it as such and expects it of a person who is placed in an intolerably embarrassing or shameful situation. Malaysian social structure emphasizes strong ties between relatives and kinfolk which result in tensions arising from these interpersonal obligations. Amok is rare (if not absent) in Malays who live in Europe and who do not have these obligations to kinfolk or among Malays in Malaysia who have left their kin groups.

Burton-Bradley summarized the cases which he had come across. They were all young men, and none had serious mental disorders (such as schizophrenia) or epilepsy.

> A healthy adult is quieter than usual or "goes bush" for a few days. There may be a history of slight or insult. He may regain his normal composure, or the condition may continue and remain unchanged (an abortive attack), or it may become worse. In this case, suddenly and without warning, without anyone expecting such an immediate response at this point of time, he jumps up, seizes an axe or some spears, rushes around attacking all and sundry and even destroying inanimate objects, such as yam houses or hospital property. Within a very short period of time, a number of people will be dead or wounded. He shouts "I am going to kill you," and everyone in the neighborhood seeks safety in flight. All are now fully aware that the man is suffering from a special form of "kava kava" or "long long" (insanity), and that he will not be satiated or stop of his own accord. They recognize that this, and other similar types of reaction, are available methods of tension reduction, used from time to time as acts arising from despair. The man continues in this fashion until overpowered, by which time he has become exhausted. He may also be killed or wounded. The attack may be aborted at any time by anyone who is brave enough to attempt it. On the subject's recovery, it is usually claimed that there is no recollection of the events that occurred during the acute phase. (1968, p. 252)

David and Gene Lester (1975) suggested that these killings may be seen as a means of delivering the person from unbearable situations. Much thinking precedes the nihilistic feeling of despair. The man sees his life as intolerable and has nothing to lose but life, and so he trades his own life for those of others. The amok episode rehabilitates him in the eyes of his group, but he runs the risk of being killed in the process. In other cases of amok, however, the man is not making a rational decision. He does lose control completely, and his strong emotions take over.

Running amok is found most commonly in Malaysia, but it has been reported in Papua and New Guinea, Trinidad, India, Liberia, Siberia, Africa, and Polynesia. It seems to be rare among the Chinese.

Joseph Westermeyer (1972, 1973) described 18 cases of amok in Laos in which the men used grenades. All the murderers were male, and 15 were soldiers. Sixteen had fathers who were farmers. The men were living away from home, drinking at the time, and 10 of them killed themselves after the attack. Most of the attacks took place at night, on weekends, in crowded places, and were a reaction to the loss (of a loved one, money or prestige).

Those who killed in these amok attacks were younger than other murderers in Laos, killed more victims, killed more often in crowded places, and more often used a grenade. They were more often living away from home and on active duty in the military, and they were more likely to have been drinking and to kill themselves after the murders than other murderers.

Ari Kiev (1972) viewed amok as a homicidal mania, but he felt that it could occur in states of delirium, agitated depression, and acute anxiety reactions. Karin Andriolo (1998) thought that the psychiatric state preceding amok was a bipolar affective disorder, what we commonly call manic-depressive psychosis. The outburst appears to be somewhat manic, and the state of exhaustion afterwards depressive, but we, the present authors, see no close correlation between manic-depressive disorder and amok, and certainly no psychiatrist has diagnosed those who run amok without already knowing about their outburst.

THE WIITIKO PSYCHOSIS[1]

According to Seymour Parker (1960), the Wiitiko psychosis is a behavior pattern found among the Algonkian-speaking Canadian-Natives in the forested central northeastern Canada, including the Saulteux, Cree, Beaver, and Ojibwa Indians. Ari Kiev (1972) viewed it as a "classic depressive disorder," but he felt that schizophrenia and manic disorder could also be involved.

[1] This is also called the Windigo psychosis.

It affects mainly males who have spent time hunting unsuccessfully for food in frozen forests. Initially the subject feels morbidly depressed and nauseated, and he experiences distaste for ordinary foods. He may have periods of semi-stupor. Gradually he becomes obsessed with the paranoidal belief that he is bewitched, and he starts having homicidal and suicidal thoughts. He feels that he is possessed by the Wiitiko monster. As the psychosis develops, he begins to see those around him as fat, luscious animals which he desires to devour. Finally, he enters a stage of violent, homicidal cannibalism. The Indians believe that if he reaches this point, he is incurable and must be killed.

There may be genetic factors, brain damage, and individually idiosyncratic traumatic experience which contribute to the "cause" of this disorder. However, Parker focused on the stress from the environment and the child-rearing techniques in the Ojibwa culture.

The Ojibwa child is at first handled permissively and indulged but, between the ages of three and five, a drastic change occurs. The child is weaned from his dependency and prodded to assume adult responsibilities. He is hardened by practices such as being made to run naked in the snow, he is goaded by the adult men to become a hunter, and he is taught by his mother how to trap animals. By age nine, he has his own hunting grounds, and by age 12 he is a competent hunter, staying away for long periods, hunting in the silent, frozen forests. The boy is made to fast until eventually he can go for long periods with only one meal a day. Punishment is often a matter of withholding food. Finally, at puberty, he is sent out into the forest without food and expected to remain there until he is able to communicate with the supernatural by means of a vision.

Parker summed up the important results of this experience as follows:

1. the period of indulgence followed by harsh weaning from dependency leads to the development of covert dependency cravings,
2. there is a close association of food, eating, and self-esteem in which to be hungry is an expression of defeat and shame,
3. power, acceptance, and affection are secured by self-denial and suffering, and
4. security and self-esteem are vulnerable and must constantly be reaffirmed by the external symbols of success.

As adults, the Ojibwa are characterized by a high level of interpersonal hostility which they express in indirect ways, hypersensitivity to insults, exaggerated pride, and a paranoid tendency.

The Ojibwa's childhood experiences lead to unsatisfied dependency cravings and repressed (unconscious) hostility. However, the social structure of Ojibwa society does not allow acceptable outlets for these needs, and the grown-up Ojibwa treads a narrow path between his quest for affection and his desire to give vent to his rage. Failure in hunting can easily lead to a psychiatric breakdown. Failure to obtain food threatens starvation and loss of self-esteem. The paranoid feelings may result from the belief that your bad luck is the result of others practicing magic against you, a belief which develops easily in those who have repressed their anger. Failure as a hunter is a stress which leads to breakdown of the normal defense mechanisms. Rage and aggression are then expressed in a direct and overt manner, rather than being turned inward as depression. In the full-blown Wiitiko psychosis, the symptoms of homicidal cannibalism serve to allay dependency cravings by becoming one with the object of dependency (by eating it) while simultaneously aggressing against this frustrating person (by killing and devouring it). The cultural belief in the Wiitiko monster symbolizes the wide circle of significant others (especially the parents) who continue to frustrate the dependency cravings of the adult and who still threaten his self-esteem.

It is notable that a mild case of Wiitiko psychosis can be treated successfully by having other people prepare a dish of melted bear grease and berries which the patient drinks. This action simultaneously lessens hunger by providing a good many calories (important in the old days when the long winters were particularly stressful for the Ojibwa), and satisfied some dependency cravings since the person is fed and cared for by others as he was when he was a child. There may also be some significance in the choice of bear grease since bears are considered by the Ojibwa to be magically important animals.

COMMENT

It can be seen that dying (and perhaps committing suicide) by getting others to kill you has been documented in many primitive societies. Suicide-by-cop, therefore, may simply be a modern version of this syndrome.

CHAPTER 6

Running Amok in America

We have seen in the previous chapter that *running amok* is found in those living in under-developed countries and in times past. Can it happen in America today?

Some commentators say, "No."

For example, Jean Baechler (1979) argued that amok must be ritualized by the culture. The culture must have a name for the phenomenon and specify the circumstances in which it is expected to occur. There must also be a typical way of running amok; that is, the sequence of behaviors and symptoms shown must be predictable.

On the other hand, many of the mass murders which have taken place in America and in other nations in recent years do seem to have a standard pattern. A man, often dressed in military fatigues, takes several guns and kills others in a manner that resembles war-time attacks. In this way, mass murder has become ritualized and has an expected course.

Dr. J. Arboleda-Florez (1979) agreed that amok can be found in modern America. He too noted that many mass murderers fit into the definition of amok quite well. There should be a brooding period, a homicidal outburst, persistent homicidal behavior without any apparent motives, and a claim of amnesia after the outburst. However, since many of the mass murderers are killed by police or commit suicide, the presence of amnesia is hard to confirm.

Arboleda-Florez described the case of a Canadian sniper who on June 16, 1977, dressed in army fatigues and carrying several guns, walked into a shopping mall in Calgary and wounded eight victims. He was captured alive, tried and convicted, and given a psychiatric evaluation by Arboleda-Florez. His memory was "hazy." He remembered going downstairs, having big pockets in his clothes (he was wearing army fatigues), going outside and feeling that the cars and people were closing in on him and that he had to shoot his way through. He felt that he was "out of himself," saw lights and colors and heard a boom. That was all.

Arboleda-Florez suggested that amok would appear in societies undergoing rapid social change. The murderer will have feelings of alienation and a need to be assertive. Arboleda-Florez thought that Charles Whitman, a mass murderer in 1966, was a classic case of amok, and so let us examine this mass murderer based on an account written by Gary Lavergne (1997).

THE MADMAN IN THE TOWER[1]

On July 31, 1966, Charles Whitman murdered his mother and his wife in Austin, Texas. The next day, he climbed the tower on the University of Texas campus and, armed with an arsenal of firearms, he killed 14 people and wounded at least 31 others. After a hour and a half, he was killed by two police officers. He was viewed by some as the "pioneer" of mass murder in the United States and by others as the American equivalent of "running amok."

Charles Whitman's father, Charles also, but known as C.A., lived in Lake Worth, Florida, a town on the Atlantic coast, with about 15,000 residents in 1955. He was a successful plumbing contractor. He met and married Margaret Hodges, who thereafter ran the office for him and kept the books. By 1963, the firm owned four cars and 21 trucks, and had 28 full-time workers. C.A. was a civic leader, president of the local Chamber of Commerce and the PTA.

He had three sons: Charles in 1941, Patrick in 1945, and John in 1949. C.A. had a bad temper and occasionally beat his wife. He was a strict disciplinarian with his sons and punished them using paddles, belts, and fists. Yet he also spoiled his family materially, moving his mother into the house next door, buying everyone in the family new cars, and the boys motorcycles as well. C.A. loved guns and introduced his boys to hunting.

Margaret was a devout Roman Catholic. She took her sons to mass regularly, and they attended parochial schools. Charlie became an altar boy and won a prize for learning Latin.

---

[1] It is important in case studies to have a detailed knowledge of the individual's whole life. Events in childhood and adolescence are critical in understanding later behavior. For example, in order to make a psychiatric diagnosis of the individuals and to classify them into a typology requires longitudinal data from the full extent of their lives. Thus, the case studies presented in this book present information about the people from birth, childhood, adolescence, and adulthood.

Charlie was born on June 24, 1941, in the doctor's office, after a normal pregnancy and delivery. He was healthy apart from the usual childhood diseases. He learned to play the piano and seemed to like that. He tried to join a band later, but C.A. forbade it. With C.A. coaching him, Charlie also became an excellent shot.

Charlie joined the cub scouts at age eight and the scouts at 11. He became the youngest eagle scout in the world at the age of 12. He earned 21 merit badges in 15 months. The scout master noticed that Charlie worked so hard in scouting because of the pressure from C.A. to excel. In grade school, Charlie was consistently on the honor roll. His IQ was measured in 1947 at 139.

Charlie took on a large paper route to earn money and, by 1955, he could afford to purchase a Harley-Davidson motor bike. In 1958, he had surgery to remove a blood clot on his left testicle.

In high school, he pitched for the baseball team and managed the football team. He was reasonably popular, but his grades dropped from 3.30 in his freshman year to 2.50 in his senior year. He graduated 7th in his class of 72. In the final two years of high school, he got five traffic tickets for problems such as accidents and double-parking.

One evening near his 18th birthday, Charlie went out with friends and came home drunk. C.A. beat him and threw him into the swimming pool, so that he almost drowned. Charlie had had enough of his father and enlisted in the Marines three days after his 18th birthday, even though he had been accepted at Georgia Tech University.

Charlie completed his basic training and was sent to Guantanamo Naval Base in Cuba in December 1959. He seemed easy-going and got the nickname "Whit." He grew to about six feet and weighed 198 pounds. He shot well-enough to be a "sharp-shooter." He earned a good conduct medal, and a medal for his service in Cuba. He then joined a scholarship program to earn a degree in engineering, after which he would become a commissioned officer. He was sent to preparatory school in Maryland in July 1961 to improve his knowledge in mathematics and physics and arrived on the University of Texas campus in September 1961. Charlie moved into the dorms and was appointed a counselor, which meant that he got free boarding.

He was soon in trouble. He and a friend poached a deer and were caught, but he was fined only $100. He was an accomplished poker player, and he occasionally paid his losses with checks that bounced. In that first year, Charlie told one of his friends:

A person could stand off an army from atop of it [the University of Texas tower] before they got to him. (Lavergne, 1997, p. 23)

Kathy Leissner was born in Needville, Texas, on July 12, 1943, and went to the University of Texas to study education. She met Charlie in February 1962. Their courtship was brief but intense. The couple was married on August 17, 1962, and went off for their honeymoon to New Orleans.

Charlie's grades his first semester were not good—A, C, D, and F. His grades improved a little after his marriage but, after a year and a half, the Marines took his scholarship away. He dropped out of the university in February 1963, and returned to Camp Lejeune, North Carolina. The Marines rejected his request for reinstatement in the college program, and he became embittered despite a promotion to Lance Corporal. He got into disciplinary problems over fighting and gambling and was court-martialled in November 1963. He turned to C.A. for help who made efforts to obtain an early discharge for Charlie, which was granted in December 1964.

During this time, Charlie started a diary in which he made resolutions for his life (such as to stop gambling) and wrote self-deprecating passages, blaming himself for his misbehavior and for the problems he caused his wife and parents.

Charlie returned to Kathy and Austin. There are indications that he was occasionally violent toward Kathy and that she feared him. He continued to gamble, but for lower stakes than in the past, and, although Kathy earned some money, they lived as poor students. Charlie changed his major from mechanical engineering to architectural engineering, and he got a job, first as a bill collector and then as a bank teller. C.A. sent them a monthly allowance and bought them a new car. They rented an apartment and then a house and got a dog named Schocie. Kathy went to a local Methodist church, and Charlie sometimes accompanied her. He also became a scout master for a few months. Colleagues noticed that he sweated a lot, even on cold days, and chewed on his fingernails. He began to put on weight and earned the nickname "Porky" from the kids.

Kathy graduated in 1965 while Charlie continued to take a full load of courses. His biographer, Gary Lavergne, thinks that Charlie could pretend to be nice, but that it was an act. He could not *be* nice. His benevolent appearance was a facade, and in his diaries he listed admonitions to himself such as don't criticize, be courteous, and be gentle to Kathy. He tried to suppress the hostility and anger he felt. He set himself goals, made lists, and labored over details. Minor setbacks discouraged him, and he seemed to achieve little. He got a real estate license in May 1965, but he never sold any properties. His lack of success and dependence on his father (plus his inability to stand up to his father) made him hate his father even more. He was also embarrassed by his father's job—cleaning cesspools.

Kathy taught for a year and then took a job part-time as an operator for the telephone company. The couple seemed to get on fine, and Charlie claimed to have hit her only twice, although they argued a lot.

In June 1966, Charlie applied for a job as an engineering laboratory assistant and proved to be a good worker. His GPA remained around 2.0, but he was liked by his fellow students and teachers and by his neighbors. Charlie now feared that he was sterile, and he began to worry that he had a brain problem.

Back home in Florida, C.A.'s relationship with his wife began to disintegrate, and Margaret left C.A. in March 1996 to go to Austin, where Margaret got herself an apartment and a job as a cashier at a cafeteria.

Charlie was now very depressed and anxious. In addition to his insecurities over his academic career and his problems with Kathy, he now had his mother to cope with and the continual calls from his father trying to enlist Charlie's help in getting Margaret back. He thought about dropping out of school and leaving Kathy. Kathy eventually persuaded Charlie to go for counseling at the university. His first session was on March 29, 1966. He was given Valium and referred to a psychiatrist. The psychiatrist, Dr. Maurice Dean Heatly, thought that Charlie was "oozing with hostility," self-centered and egocentric, but also motivated to improve himself. Charlie admitted he wanted to be superior to his father. He mentioned that he had thoughts of going up the tower on campus with a deer rifle and shooting people.

In 1966, Charlie visited the tower on the campus several times, once with his younger brother, John. The tower rose 307 feet above the campus and had an observation deck on the 28th floor circling the tower, 231 feet above ground level.

Charlie began to take amphetamines, especially when studying for final exams. The drugs led to mood swings and insomnia, so he took Librium to go to sleep. He also took Excedrin for his headaches. In July, Charlie, his younger brother John, and Kathy went for a brief visit to San Antonio. Charlie also signed up for 14 semester hours of summer school as well as continuing to work as a laboratory assistant. The weather in Austin was close to 100° all month.

The last week in July seemed uneventful for Charlie and Kathy. People who saw Charlie on July 31 described him as calm. That Sunday, at 6.45 P.M., Charlie typed a suicide note. He described his stress and his lack of understanding of himself and of his violent impulses. He asked for an autopsy after his death to see if he had a physical disorder. A tumor was found in his brain upon autopsy, but the pathologist thought it was not the cause of Whitman's rampage. He wrote that he planned to kill his wife after he picked her up from work, even though he loved her dearly. He did not want her to suffer in the world as he had. Friends interrupted his typing, and they went out to buy some ice cream.

THE MURDERS

Charlie picked up Kathy at 9.30 P.M. and drove her home. Charlie then went over to his mother's apartment while Kathy went to bed to sleep. He arrived at his mother's apartment just after midnight. He probably strangled her from behind with a rubber hose, damaged the back of her head either with a blow or a shotgun (no autopsy was performed), crushed her left hand, and stabbed her in the chest. He then sat down and wrote a note saying that he loved his mother and wanted to spare her more suffering. He also expressed his rage toward his father. He placed his mother in her bed as if she were asleep.

Charlie got home around 2.30 A.M. and stabbed his sleeping wife to death with five blows to the chest. He then finished his suicide note. For the next seven hours, Charlie got ready for the slaughter. He made lists and purchased and accumulated weapons and supplies for a long siege (of several days), including such items as an alarm clock and food as well as guns, ammunition, and knives. He called Kathy's and Margaret's supervisors to say that they were ill and would not be in for work. Having purchased his supplies and additional guns, he put on overalls to seem like a repairman, loaded his car with his supplies and drove to the campus at 11.00 A.M.

He got a permit from the campus guard to unload equipment, drove to the tower, loaded up a dolly, and entered the tower. He went up to the 27th floor and climbed the steps to the 28th floor. He killed the receptionist, Edna Townsley, immediately with blows to the head and dragged her out of sight. (He later shot her in the head.) Just then, two visitors to the tower came through to go down, and Charlie simply smiled at them and let them pass. Soon after this, two families came up to the observation deck, the Gabours and the Lamberts—two wives, two husbands, and two sons. Charlie opened fire on them and then barricaded the doors. One son and one wife were killed immediately, the other son and wife were injured, while the two men (coming up last) escaped injury.

It was now 11:48 A.M., and the observation deck was secured.

For the next hour and a half, Charlie shot people around the campus, in a five-block area, mostly with his 6mm Remington with a four-power scope. Some were killed instantaneously, others were wounded. Rescue of the wounded was made difficult since Charlie shot at would-be rescuers. Some of the wounded lay for hours on the ground, suffering from burns as a result of extreme heat. The local emergency rooms received 39 victims, 12 dead or soon to die.

As the news spread, police and armed citizens poured in to the campus. They suspected that several men were up on the tower shooting, and it was not until the end that they realized that there was only one man up there. As Charlie moved around that observation deck, dozens of police and civilians, side-by-side, fired their pistols, rifles, and shotguns toward the tower. Charlie hit most of his victims in the first 15 minutes because thereafter he had to duck and move to avoid being hit himself.

Eventually, police entered the tower, and Houston McCoy, a three-year member of the Austin Police Department, and Ramiro Martinez, a five-year veteran, made it to the observation deck, along with a civilian, Allen Crum, and two other police officers, Jerry Day and Phillip Conner.

Martinez and McCoy crawled around the deck, eventually encountering Charlie. Martinez saw Charlie first and shot six rounds from his revolver as fast as he could. McCoy followed and fired his shotgun twice. Martinez grabbed the shotgun after McCoy reloaded and ran toward Charlie, firing again. Charlie was dead at 1:24 P.M.

McCoy felt that Whitman could have shot them both, but that he was waiting for them and wanted to be shot.

This style of mass murder, later called *pseudo-commando,* seemed to become the model for mass murder, not simply in America, but also elsewhere. Similar incidents later occurred in England and Australia. The incidents are different from "running amok" in that the pseudo-commandos often have planned their killings carefully and seem calm as they pick off their victims. In contrast, those who run amok in less developed nations seem more impulsive and more frantic in their killing.

It is interesting to note, of course, that in this first modern mass murder, Charlie expected to die. He wrote his suicide note before leaving to commit his first murder (that of his mother). It is not clear whether he planned to commit suicide himself or whether he anticipated that the police would shoot him. But it is clear that he intended to commit suicide one way or another!

CHAPTER 7
Victim-Precipitated Murder

When murders are investigated, it is frequently found that the victim has played an important part in bringing about his own death. He has, in a sense, committed suicide, using another person as his weapon. Marvin Wolfgang (1958, 1959) some 40 years ago called this behavior *victim-precipitated homicide*.

The proportion of victim-precipitated homicides is startling. In his study of 588 homicides which occurred in Philadelphia between 1948 and 1952, Wolfgang found that 160 (26%) of them had occurred after direct provocation by the victim. In many cases, the victim started the quarrel or was the first to show or use a weapon.

> For example, a husband had threatened to kill his wife during several violent family quarrels. He would usually later admit his regret for having beaten her and for having suggested the idea of her death. In the last instance, he first attacked her with a pair of scissors, dropped them, and then grabbed a butcher knife from the kitchen. In the ensuing struggle, which ended on their bed, she had possession of the knife, and there was considerable doubt in the minds of the jury whether the husband invited his wife to stab him or deliberately fell on the knife. In another case, a drunken husband, beating his wife in their kitchen, gave her a butcher knife and dared her to use it on him. She claimed that if he should strike her once more she would use the knife, whereupon he slapped her in the face and she fulfilled the promise he apparently expected by fatally stabbing him. (Wolfgang, 1958, p. 92)

What sort of victim precipitates his own murder? He differs from the murder victim who is judged not to have provoked his own murder, and he is also different from the person who simply kills himself. For example, in Wolfgang's study about 80 percent of the victims who precipitated their own murders were black, while blacks made up only

70 percent of the victims of ordinary murders. A larger difference is apparent when murder victims are compared to suicides: only 10 percent of those dying by suicide were black.

A large majority (94%) of the victims who provoked homicide were men. The majority of deaths from ordinary murder and from suicide were those of men too, but the proportions were smaller: 70 percent and 77 percent, respectively. The murderer was much more likely to be a woman in a victim-precipitated homicide (29%) than in ordinary murders (14%).

Victims who precipitated their own murder were more likely to have been drinking than victims who did not provoke the act. Perhaps the influence of alcohol played a role in the victim's provocative behavior. Excessive drinking can itself be seen as a self-destructive behavior (Karl Menninger [1938] called it "chronic suicide" since excessive alcohol use shortens one's life), and this is in character with provoking your own murder. Alternatively, it may be that the effects of alcohol prevented the victim from defending himself as he might otherwise had done had he been sober.

Precipitation of the murder by the victim was more common in slayings of spouses. In the victim-precipitated deaths, 22 percent involved spouses, while only 15 percent of other murders involved spouses. When the murder of a spouse was precipitated by the victim, the dead person was the husband rather than the wife in 85 percent of the cases. The husband was killed in a much smaller number of the spouse murders which were not victim-precipitated, only 28 percent. Perhaps this is the case because a man can threaten physical violence to his wife or actively harm her, frightening her into killing him, more easily than a wife can do so to her husband.

Wolfgang speculated that a husband who provokes his wife to kill him has unconsciously selected a mother substitute as the agent of death. He thought that this might have some relevance to the higher proportion of blacks involved in victim-precipitated homicide, since it has been suggested that the mother in black families is a more important figure than the mother in a white family.

Police records show that victims who precipitated their own murders had been arrested more often than those who did not. This was true even when crimes of assault alone were considered. In contrast, the killers who were provoked by their victims were less likely to have been arrested than those who killed spontaneously.

The victim who provokes his murderer is more likely to belong to the lower than the upper socioeconomic classes. Wolfgang thought that assaultive behavior is more socially acceptable and more common in lower-class than in middle-class or upper-class groups. He suggested that the kinds of aggressive acts to which a person is accustomed affect his ideas of culturally appropriate or culturally acceptable ways to die.

Wolfgang noted that physical aggression is more common in the lower classes (lower class parents are, for example, more likely to punish their children physically), and the longer arrest records suggested to him a less well-developed conscience. Since murder is more common in the lower classes, and suicide less common, the lower class subculture socializes the individual into expressing his aggression more outwardly and less inwardly. Murder is probably seen as a "masculine" behavior while suicide is viewed as a "feminine" behavior.

The victim-precipitated murderer both aggresses outwardly (toward the person he provokes into murdering him) and inwardly (by getting this other person to punish by means of murder). Perhaps he feels guilty for past assaultive behavior and other misdeeds. His desires to murder and to be punished are both satisfied. Whereas middle class people have internalized cultural norms (and so feel guilty and atone for their misdeeds), lower class people seek restraint and direction from external sources. In choosing a wife to be his murderer, Wolfgang speculated that the man is selecting a mother-figure as his murderer and so is in a symbolic, but unconscious, child-parent relationship with his murderer.

For lower class black men, in particular, suicide may be seen as an "unmanly" and "weak" death, while dying in a fight may be considered to be an admirable way to die. When the individual wants to die (presumably because of pressures which might lead to suicide in a member of another group), he may unconsciously seek out a potential murderer and behave so aggressively that he is killed.

With reference to the idea of victim-precipitated homicide as a form of suicide, such a death is a particularly hostile form of committing suicide. It has been hypothesized that some suicidal acts are a way of expressing rage. This would seem to be especially true of victim-precipitated homicide. First, the victim-to-be shows his anger in the initial provocation of a potential murderer. Second, if a fight occurs prior to the murder, aggressive impulses can be expressed through the blows. Finally, although the victim is probably not consciously aware of the fact, his choice of death almost guarantees that the murderer will be punished by the criminal justice system and perhaps be tortured by guilt over killing him.

William Foote (1999) has looked at the research done on victim-precipitated murder (VPH) since Wolfgang's early study. In Chicago, one study found that 37 percent of the murders were victim-precipitated. In this study, the victims of victim-precipitated murders were older than the victims of ordinary murders. As in

Wolfgang's study, most of the victims of VPH were male (89%). In a second study, 81 percent of husbands killed by wives were VPH as compared to only 10 percent of wives killed by husbands. Domestic quarrels seem to lead to VPH more often than they lead to ordinary murder, and VPH participants seem to be intoxicated more often than those involved in ordinary murders. Stabbing is more often the method for VPH murder, but this may result from more of the murderers being women.

Foote suggested that all VPH victims tend to be risk-takers and aggressive. They can be distinguished, however, in terms of the intentionality of their provocative behavior. Foote called the obviously provocative VPH victim a *hetero-suicide*. They choose potential murderers who are bigger and have more fighting experience and who are better armed. Suicide-by-cop would fit into this category.

These victims show a clear desire to die, engage in premeditation and planning, give the killer no choice but to kill him, and may commit a serious crime in order to increase the chances of being killed. Foote speculated that these individuals may show signs of grandiosity (thinking that they are especially smart) and paranoia (thinking that others are out to get them). They may see themselves as victims and seek a situation that confirms this view.

Less obvious VPH are those individuals who continually place themselves in death-likely situations, such as those who regularly drink heavily at bars, late into the night, and who often get into fights with other bar patrons. Foote called these people "Dangerous people in dangerous places." Moving along the continuum from VPH to less precipitation, Foote next described the assaultive spouse, who runs the risk that, one day, his battered wife may turn on him. And finally, Foote described the thief who runs the risk of being killed by the shopkeepers or homeowners he tries to rob.

William Foote suggested that preventing the victim of VPH from being murdered involves:

- helping to relieve his depression,
- treating his alcohol and drug addiction, if present,
- prescribing anti-psychotic medication to reduce the paranoia and grandiosity,
- hospitalizing the person if the risk seems great, especially if the potential victim of VPH has experienced an interpersonal loss, and
- getting the family into therapy if the potential murderer and victim are family members.

CHAPTER 8

Suicide at the Hands of the State

Jean Baechler (1979) suggested that the term *indirect suicide* could be used to label the victim-precipitated suicides described in the previous chapter—behavior that is designed to provoke a homicidal reaction in another person. Baechler gave an example from the 7th century. A married priest, Petros of Kapitolion (in the province of Damascus in Syria), liked the idea of becoming a martyr. To achieve this, he made a series of comments that offended the Muslims who ruled the region in which he lived. (He may have been trying to convert Muslims to Christianity.) Although the Muslim rulers were remarkably tolerant,[1] he eventually forced them to execute him.

Some martyrs may be seen as motivated in part by suicidal desires, although, of course, many other motives may also be present. In a discussion of martyrs in the Ottoman Empire in the 15th through 19th centuries, Demetrios Constantelos (1978) noted many reasons for martyrdom, including political protest and social agitation, atonement for converting to Islam, and imitation of earlier martyrs. For example, Romanos from central Greece went on a pilgrimage to Jerusalem and was inspired by listening to the Acts of the Martyrs read in the monastery there to become a martyr, and he succeeded in getting himself executed in 1694.

It has been suggested that some murderers are trying to commit suicide, perhaps unconsciously, by getting the state to execute them, at least in countries where the death penalty is in force. For example, Theodore Dorpat (1968) noted that Lee Harvey Oswald, the presumed assassin of President John F. Kennedy, left many clues to his identity, including fingerprints on the rifle. He also brought attention to himself by going to a movie after the crime and shooting a police officer who approached him.

[1] They labeled him as mad in order to spare him.

It has been observed that some inmates on death row eventually volunteer to give in to the process leading to their execution. They stop all appeals and accept the death sentence. However, it is by no means clear that they felt this way before their crime or immediately after conviction.

David Lester (1998b) has calculated the suicide rate on death row in the United States. The rate was 146 per 100,000 per year (the usual way of calculating suicide rates) as compared to only 25 per 100,000 per year in prison inmates in general. This high suicide rate on death row is remarkable because inmates there are more closely supervised than in other parts of those prisons and in other prisons.

Baechler provided the example of a French murderer, Claude Buffet, who had demanded the death penalty, but who was instead sentenced to life imprisonment. Buffet then tried to escape, taking hostages, and killed two of these in order force the authorities to execute him, which they did in December 1972. Buffet had reasoned that, since the Christian religion forbids suicide, the only way to exit this life prematurely and without sinning was to be killed. Buffet wrote to the French President, "To kill in order to commit suicide, that's my morality" (Baechler, 1979, p. 36). Baechler cites a French report that identified 28 such murderers in France.

Robert Hughes (1986), in his history of Australia, noted that in the early 1800s, Australian authorities sent their worst criminals to Norfolk Island, 1,000 miles offshore in the Pacific Ocean, where conditions were horrendous. One way of committing suicide went as follows. A group of men would draw straws to select two of their number. These two would then draw straws to choose who would kill the other. Thus, one of the men would escape Norfolk Island by death. The murderer would then have to be shipped back to Sydney on the mainland for trial. This gave the man a slim chance for escape. If he failed to escape, then he would be tried, convicted of murder, and hung. Thus, the second man would escape Norfolk Island, most probably by being executed by the state.

Several classic cases of this type occurred in olden times.

CLASSIC CASES

Antigone

Oedipus is famous for inadvertently murdering his father (he did not know the identity of his victim) and then marrying his mother (again unknowingly). When he discovered the reality of his actions, his mother/wife committed suicide, and he blinded himself. He eventually died, leaving four children. Eteocles allied himself with the new king, Creon, while the other son, Polynices led a rebellion and lost. Both brothers were killed in the civil war.

Their sister Antigone then has lost her mother, Jocasta, many years ago, and now her father/brother, Oedipus. Her brothers have fought each other, and both are dead. She has suffered great loss.

Antigone decides to bury her brother Polynices against Creon's orders, knowing that the punishment is to be stoned to death. After failing to persuade her sister Ismene to assist her, she asks Ismene to tell everyone what she is going to do. Her first attempt to bury her brother is discovered, and he is unburied. When she buries him a second time, she "screamed like an angry bird" (Sophocles, 1956, p. 137) so as to be sure to get caught.

Having been caught, Antigone refuses now to let Ismene share the blame (and the glory):

> You chose; life was your choice, when mine was death. (Sophocles, 1956, p. 141)

and, rather than trying to placate Creon, she angrily attacks him, goading him into sentencing her to death—truly a victim-precipitated homicide.

Antigone anticipates a public death, and she compares herself with the death of the daughter of Tantalus. The Chorus then reminds Antigone that Tantalus's daughter (Niobe) was a goddess, while Antigone is a mere mortal, which upsets Antigone:

> Mockery, mockery! By the gods of our fathers,
> Must you make me a laughing stock while I yet live?
> (Sophocles, 1956, p. 149)

However, Creon orders Antigone to be sealed in a cave, rather than being killed in public. Antigone hangs herself (using the same method for suicide as did her mother) after being placed in the cave.

But Antigone does not anticipate joining her fiancé Haemon.

> So to my grave,
> My bridal bower . . .
> O but I would not have done the forbidden thing
> For any husband or for any son.
> For why? I could have another husband
> And by him other sons, if one were lost;
> But . . . where would I get
> Another brother?
> (Sophocles, 1956, p. 150)

It is Polynices who has Antigone's affection. In her death, her bridal-bower, as she calls it, it is Polynices with whom she looks forward to being reunited—implications of an incestuous desire with a brother who, as is common in such incestuous situations between brothers and sisters, has been away from Antigone for most of their childhood and adolescence.

In her death, Antigone succeeds in transforming her image. The child of an incestuous marriage, she defies Creon and dies heroically, leaving Creon cast as the villain. She commits suicide by getting Creon to execute her. Only when she is deprived of her public execution, a victim-precipitated homicide, does she hang herself.

Socrates

Socrates was the son of Sophroniscus and Phaenarete from Alopeke, a town on the road from Athens to the marble quarries of Pentelicon. He was born in 470 B.C. or 469 B.C. He was executed in 399 B.C. at the age of 70.

His father has been described as a stonemason and as a sculptor, and Socrates may have learned the craft as a youth before he became a philosopher/teacher. His mother was perhaps a midwife. As a young man, he participated in the Peloponnesian War between Sparta and Athens which was won by Sparta. He was obviously noteworthy in Athens since Aristophanes and Ameipsias both made him the subject of comedies in 423 B.C.

He next appeared in the historical record in 406 B.C. when it was his turn to participate in the Council of Five Hundred, and he argued against trying the generals at the battle of Arginusae as a group—such a trial was in fact illegal under Athenian law.

He married late in life to Xanthippe, by whom he had three sons, one still an infant when Socrates died. His wife has been described as a shrew, but some commentators have suggested it was far from easy being the wife of an old philosopher who earned no money and appeared rather indifferent to his family. (Socrates lived on income from a small inheritance from his father.)

Socrates was quite ugly, with a broad, flat, turned-up nose, prominent staring eyes, thick fleshy lips, and a paunch. He regularly went about barefoot, wearing an old coat, and unwashed. He was considered to have excellent self-control. He was never drunk, and he kept his appetite for food and sex under strict control.

Socrates was put on trial in 399 B.C., found guilty, and sentenced to death. The traditional death sentence in Athens was to drink hemlock, but what makes Socrates' death a suicide was not simply his acquiescence to the death sentence, but the fact that he could easily have escaped a guilty verdict and the death sentence. According to a recent biographer, I. F. Stone (1988), he sought to be executed, and this is what makes his death truly suicidal!

Athens was a fully participatory democracy with freedom of speech as one of its main tenets. As a result, Athens attracted thinkers from all over who came there to exchange ideas and to debate one another. Socrates was one of the leading philosophers there, but his views were rather odd. First, Socrates was completely opposed to democracy. He favored authoritarian rule by experts. Just as shoemakers must know how to make shoes, rulers must know how to rule. Only those who have the correct knowledge should be allowed to rule. Then the ruler orders, and the ruled must obey. Clearly, Socrates and his followers were out of step with the Athenians.

Did Socrates threaten the leaders of Athens? Socrates used his wisdom to make the leaders appear to be ignorant fools and, by his tactics, he turned some of the young men of the city against the democracy and encouraged them to hold even the common people of Athens in disdain. However, the playwrights frequently did this in their plays, and they were not censored, so this in itself is not sufficient cause for the trial of Socrates.

Athens was based on participation by all in the government of the city, while Socrates preached withdrawal from political life. For himself, in 70 years, he hardly participated. Although he did not participate in either of the two movements which overthrew the democracy, neither did he participate in the restoration of democracy.

Important for understanding the reasons for his trial and conviction was the fact that two of his students helped overthrow the democratic government in Athens. Part of the charge against Socrates was that he led the youth to despise the established constitution and made them violent. In 411 B.C. the overthrow of the government was led by Alcibiades after which followed a period of rule by the Four Hundred. In 404 B.C., a group of 30 overthrew the government, aided by Sparta which had defeated Athens in the Peloponnesian War.

The rule of the Four Hundred lasted only four months and the rule of Thirty only eight months, but there were many horrors committed during those brief periods. The possibility of new horrors must have scared the Athenians so much that Socrates's ideas were now seen as very dangerous. In both coups, the aristocracy joined with the middle classes to disfranchise the lower classes, and then the aristocracy turned against the middle class. The aristocracy proved to be cruel, rapacious, and bloody. The Thirty killed more than 1,500

Athenians in eight months, more than had died in the last decade of the Peloponnesian War.

Although there was an amnesty after the coup of 404 B.C., some of the Thirty refused to be reconciled and moved to the nearby town of Eleusis. The Athenians learned that the leaders of Eleusis were planning to attack Athens in 401 B.C. and attacked first and defeated them. Thus, Athens in 399 B.C. had much to fear from the followers of Socrates, and so they tried him.

Stone estimated that the vote for Socrates' guilt was probably 280 for conviction and 220 for acquittal. Socrates was surprised that so many voted for acquittal for, according to Xenophon, he did his best to antagonize the jury, particularly by being boastful and arrogant. It seemed as if 70 years of life was enough for Socrates, and he was worried about becoming frail and losing his hearing and vision. He acknowledged that trial and execution was a way to commit suicide, what we now call a *victim-precipitated homicide,* because the victim acts in such a way as to force (or encourage) others kill him.

Next came the vote for the penalty. Athenian juries could vote only for the penalty proposed by the prosecution or that proposed by the accused. The prosecution demanded the death penalty. Socrates offered first that he should be fed free of charge for the rest of his life as a civic hero. He next offered a fine of one mina, a trivial amount but, following pressure from Plato and other followers, suggested 30 minas of silver. The jury voted for the death penalty by a vote of about 360 to 140.

A proposal of banishment from the city or a reasonable fine would have pleased the jury. He probably could have won acquittal by appealing to the Athenian commitment to free speech. But for Socrates to appeal to the Athenian system would have given the system a moral victory over him.

After the verdict, when Socrates was in prison, his followers arranged for his escape. Socrates refused. He said it was his duty to obey the court's verdict and die. So Socrates drank the hemlock that was provided to him by the court and died and, in doing so, fulfilled his own death wish.

MODERN CASES

A number of authors have described more recent cases. Frederic Wertham (1949) described the case of a patient he had seen in psychotherapy, Robert Irwin, who had mentioned early in 1931 that he had thought of killing his girl-friend in order to be executed by the state. In 1937, he tried to kill an ex-girl-friend but, because she was not living at home, he killed her mother and sister and a boarder instead, after which he gave himself up to the police. (Incidentally, he was not executed. He was sentenced to 139 years in prison.)

Thorsten Sellin (1959) described many such cases from the 1700s and 1800s and noted that they must have been quite common since the Danish government decided in 1767 to waive the death penalty in cases where the offender murdered in order to be executed. Sellin mentioned two cases from the 1900s: a Frenchman, unable to kill himself, who stabbed a woman unknown to him in order to be executed by the state, and Federick Field, who killed two people in London in 1931 in order to be executed.

More recently, Robert Bohm (1999) described the case of Daniel Colwell who was sentenced to die in the electric chair in Georgia in 1998. Colwell confessed that he was unable to kill himself, and so he shot two strangers in a parking lot so that the state would execute him. He later changed his mind and began appealing the death sentence.

Katherine van Wormer (1995) presented summaries of 20 such cases that she had located in both recent scholarly and newspaper articles on the death penalty, and one of the cases she summarized was that of Gary Gilmore.

Gary Gilmore

Gary Gilmore was executed in Utah in 1977 for the murder of two men during the commission of armed robberies. No one had been executed in America for the prior 10 years, a period during which the United States Supreme Court deliberated the conditions under which executions were permissible under the Constitution.

More than most recent murderers, Gilmore seemed to want to be executed. Indeed, he insisted upon his execution, and he seemed to be saying that state could not punish him because he desired to die by execution. The state apparently would help him in his final act of murder—that of himself. Perhaps also, although this is less clear, Gilmore murdered the men during armed robberies in part in order to ensure his execution.

His Parents

Bessie Brown was a Mormon, and her son, Mikal Gilmore (1994), who wrote about Gary Gilmore and the family, saw the Mormons as steeped in murder. Initially persecuted through the burning of their farms, the rape of their women, and the murder of their men, including the murder of their leader Joseph Smith, they migrated to Utah to escape the persecution. However, once there, they became the persecutors, following their own rule that blood must be atoned by blood. Their police force and avengers murdered many residents, and in 1857 slaughtered a group of emigrants from Arkansas passing through the state.

Bessie was born August 19, 1913, the fourth child of nine on a small farm in Provo, Utah. Bessie hated farm life as well as her father, who was physically abusive to his children, particularly Bessie and her older brother George. Bessie remembered her father taking her to a public hanging and forcing her to watch it, although Mikal could find no record of a public hanging at that time.

Bessie moved to Salt Lake City in the mid 1930s with three friends, at first working as a housekeeper. In 1936 she disappeared, perhaps hitchhiking to California and falling in love, but returning to Utah when the romance soured. In the summer of 1937, back in Salt Lake City, Bessie met Frank Gilmore, the ex-boyfriend of her best friend. Frank sold ads for *Utah Magazine,* he said, but he soon got married to another woman. Bessie ran into Frank a year later, by which time he was divorced! He proposed to Bessie, and she accepted.

Frank said that he had been a clown and performer for Barnum & Bailey Circus and a stuntman in Hollywood. He was 47 years old, Bessie was 18. They were married unofficially in Sacramento by Frank's mother, Fay, a licensed minister in the Spiritualist Church of California. They stayed with Fay for a while, and there they met Robert Ingram, 19 years old, a son of Frank by an earlier marriage. It turned out that Bessie was Frank's sixth or seventh wife and that Frank had half a dozen children scattered over the nation. Fay believed that Frank always legitimately married and divorced the wives.

Frank was led to believe by his mother that his real father was the famous magician Harry Houdini, but Mikal does not believe that this was true. He was born on November 23, 1890, while Fay was married to Harry Gilmore. Fay divorced Harry a year later, and she sent her son Frank off to boarding schools. Frank, therefore, grew up without a father and was rarely with his mother.

After Bessie and Frank's marriage, Frank began to go off on business for weeks at a time, telling Bessie nothing about what he did. They did visit Bessie's parents who disliked Frank. Bessie's father was convinced that Frank had spent time in prison. Soon after that, Frank and Bessie began wandering across America from town to town. Frank's career involved scamming. He moved to a town, sold the businessmen ads for a nonexistent magazine, and then moved on with their money. Frank also seemed to be running from something, some event and its consequences that Bessie did not know. Eventually she did find out and she told it to her son, Gary, but they never told anyone else.

Their first child, Frank Jr., was born in 1939 in Los Angeles. Gary was born in 1940 in Texas, on a cross-country trip, under an alias. Frank had signed in as Coffman and named Gary "Fay Robert Coffman." After they left Texas, they tore up the birth certificate and renamed him Gary. However, later in his life, Gary found out that his real name was indeed Fay Robert Coffman, and he came to believe that Frank was not his real father. Frank was in fact his real father, but Mikal eventually found out that Frank Jr. was fathered by Frank's son Robert while Frank himself was away on business. Yet Frank himself thought that Gary was the son of Robert!

Frank abused Bessie physically and, for several years, life continued in this way, the two of them traveling around America with two babies, fighting all the time. One day in Missouri, after a row, Frank drove off with Gary, abandoning Bessie and Frank Jr. Bessie's parents wired her bus fare to get home to Provo where she received a call from an orphanage in Iowa telling her that Gary had been dropped off there after Frank had been jailed for passing a bad check. Frank came back to Utah after he was released, and they took off again.

Frank was arrested next in December 1941, in Colorado, and Bessie found out that his criminal record went all the way back to 1914. Frank was sentenced to five years in prison, and Bessie went home to Provo. Her parents made her stay in a shack, and Bessie began to abuse the two children. Her parents threatened to take the children away from her, but Frank got out of prison after 18 months and took his family away. Frank had now become even meaner than he was.

A third son, Gaylen, was born on December 12, 1944, and he quickly became Frank's favorite. The nomadic existence continued for the rest of the 1940s. Bessie had to live with little money, a drunken husband, and three kids. They often slept in flophouses, Salvation Army shelters, and missions for vagrants. Frank continued to disappear for days at a time.

In 1946, Frank's mother Fay died, and he had a hard time adjusting. He cried, quit working, and drank heavily. A doctor who was called in told him he would be dead in a couple of years if he did not stop drinking, and surprisingly he stopped, with only occasional lapses in the following years. However, he had been meaner to his sons when sober than when drunk, and so he now became even more brutal toward them and Bessie. Bessie fought back, and fights during meals were commonplace.

At this time, Gary started having nightmares in which he was being beheaded. He had trouble sleeping, and he often wet the bed.

Frank became disenchanted with wandering, and in 1948 the family settled in Portland, Oregon, where they bought a house. When he next suggested moving, Bessie refused, and so they stayed. Bessie also persuaded Frank to actually produce a book or magazine, and in 1949 Frank produced his first *Building Codes Digest,* summarizing the codes of the region, for which he also sold advertising.

Bessie had a fourth baby a year or two after Gaylen, but he lived only a few days. Bessie and Frank decided to try for one more child and Michael, who later changed his name to Mikal, was born February 9, 1951. Soon afterwards, Bessie decided that Michael was odd, and Frank found her about to suffocate the new baby. Thereafter, Mikal became Frank's favorite, and Frank protected him from Bessie. Although he continued to be brutal toward the three older sons, Mikal was beaten only once.

Bessie and Frank finally married legally, under their real names, on June 7, 1951, in Elko, Nevada.

Gary's Life

In 1951, the family moved to Salt Lake City, and Gary (and Frank Jr.) missed their friends in Portland. Gary made friends with a new crowd, who smoked, stole, and talked about guns. Gary was found playing Russian Roulette with a gun (unloaded, he claimed) and got into physical fights with neighbors. Gary began to steal—cookies, comic books, and small toys mostly.

In early 1952, the family moved back to Portland, where they found that the neighbor to whom they had given Gary's dog had just had her put to sleep after the dog attacked her.

Instead of spankings, Frank now fiercely beat his older sons—with razor straps, belts, and bare fists—almost weekly. Soon a pattern developed, in which Bessie would intervene and then Frank and Bessie would fight. Frank Jr. tried hard not to scream or cry during the beatings, and Frank would let up. Gary could not stop screaming and so was beaten worse.

In later years, when in prison, Gary would challenge the guards who would then beat him. Still he would spit at them and call them names, bringing on more beatings, as if he was reliving the beatings from his father but handling them in a better fashion than he had as a kid. He once told his uncle that his father was the first person he really hated and that, if he could have gotten away with it, he would have killed him.

The 1950s was when rock-and-roll was popular and juvenile delinquency increased in frequency. Gary and Gaylen joined both movements. They dressed in motorcycle jackets and boots, smoked, drank alcohol and cough syrup, skipped school, and tried to make out with girls.

Gary finished grammar school at the local Catholic school and moved to the Joseph Lane Grade School, a school with mainly working-class kids. One teacher there, Tom Lyden, remembered Gary as quiet, intelligent, and with artistic talent. But Gary soon began to act up and cause trouble—sleeping, showing off, and insulting teachers. Years later, Gary remembered Lyden as the teacher he respected and liked, but at the time Lyden failed to reach Gary and divert him from his path.

If Gary could not be respected, he wanted to be feared. He drank whiskey, took nude photos of his girl-friends, and stood on the railroad tracks as trains approached until the last possible moment. He began a paper route simply to check out homes to burglarize. He began to break and enter at the age of 12 or 13. In October 1954, he broke into a gun store and stole a Winchester rifle and cartridges. That year, he also ran away from home and was picked up in Burley, Idaho. In the summer of 1955, he and some friends vandalized his school, but Frank hired a good lawyer to get him off.

In February 1955, his parents let Gary quit high school and hitchhike to Texas with some friends. Back home, they began stealing cars at night and returning them in the morning. The courts gave Gary warnings at first but, after stealing a 1948 Chevrolet, Gary was sent to MacLaren's Reform School in Woodburn, Oregon. He went in as a unruly 15-year-old; he came out after a year committed to a criminal career. While there, he tried to escape and was frequently violent, and he was beaten, locked up in isolation, and probably sexually abused. He spent most of the time being punished and, indeed, came to prefer the isolation in the maximum security unit. He earned a reputation of being very tough and frightening, but by June 1956, Gary seemed to have changed. He began to discuss his problems more with the counselors, and they decided that he should be paroled, attend high school, seek part-time work, and avoid his delinquent friends. He was released on September 1, 1955.

Back home, the fights with his father continued, and Frank refused to pay for Gary's continued counseling. Gary went back to breaking and entering, looking for money, drugs, and guns. One night he stole $18,000 from a supermarket. He got a year's probation for stealing a car, and he accidentally shot his friend after burglarizing another store. His friend refused to press charges, but Gary was sentenced in adult court to a year in the county jail. He was now 16.

He was discharged in May 1958, and went back to working a little by day and a life of crime in the evenings. Eventually, the family of an under-age girl he had slept with pressed charges, and Gary was arrested for statutory rape. He escaped from the police station and fled to California and Texas, where he was picked up for vagrancy and sent back to Oregon. The rape charge was dropped after the girl had a son and Frank agreed to pay child support. But Gary was charged with car theft and sent to the Oregon State Correctional Facility in September 1960. It was there that the authorities found out about his original name and told Gary, after which Gary came to believe that Frank was not his real father. Gary now began to have migraine headaches which bothered him for the rest of life. Gary returned home in the fall of 1961, now 21, and, according to Frank Jr., much meaner than ever before.

Gary began to use drugs more often—uppers, grass, cough syrup, heroin, and alcohol. He told Frank Jr. that he missed jail, where his real friends were. If he didn't get back, he said, he would eventually hurt someone; in fact he probably would do so in order to get back.

Frank got cancer in 1962, and Gary cried when he heard the news. Frank died later that year while Gary was in jail in Washington state after being arrested for driving without a license and with alcohol in the car. When the guards told Gary that his father had died, Gary tore his cell apart and slashed his wrists with a broken light bulb.

Gary was released after six months and hung out with his brother Gaylen, robbing, drinking, and having sex orgies. Gary made friends with people who dealt drugs and ran prostitutes, and he earned a reputation as a reliable and tough back-up man. He spent brief periods in jail where he acted crazy at times. He claimed that the soup was poisoned and that there was radar installed, and he set fires in his cell. The jail psychiatrist thought at first he was simply trying to get transferred to a psychiatric ward where life would be easier but, after slashing his wrists, Gary was transferred.

Gary next committed an armed robbery with a friend and assaulted other inmates in the jail while awaiting trial. He continued to cut himself. Gary told the doctors that he wanted to die, to bleed to death. He was diagnosed as a sociopathic personality, antisocial type, with intermittent psychotic decompensation.

He was tried in March 1964, and sentenced to 15 years in the Oregon State Penitentiary. The prison had a riot in 1968 in which Gary took part, and Mikal heard that Gary stabbed a man who had hurt one of Gary's friends and beat one man so badly that he lived the rest of his life as a "vegetable."

In prison, Gary's teeth deteriorated, and he had them extracted. The dentures were a poor fit, and Gary argued with the prison authorities about this for years. (Only in 1975, when he was transferred to the federal prison in Marion, Illinois, did he get a good set of dentures.) He fought with guards and other prisoners and was often isolated as a punishment, and he set fires. In 1971, the prison put Gary on prolixin to control his behavior, but his reactions to the drug were so bad that they took him off it. After this, his hatred of the prison authorities increased further, and his battles with them intensified, no matter what the consequences were for Gary.

In late 1971, Gaylen died from stab wounds he had received many months earlier in a fight. Bessie went to the prison to tell Gary, who cried at the news. After this, Gary changed a little. He began to write to Mikal, and the prison allowed Gary home visits under supervision (by an armed guard). He painted in prison and won some art contests. The authorities decided to parole him to a halfway house in Eugene, Oregon, on condition that he attended community college and got good grades. He tried to enroll, but he was intimidated by the procedures and did not do so. He then left the halfway house. He was arrested for armed robbery of a service station, tried in February 1973, and sentenced to nine years, despite a reasoned plea from Gary that prison would not help and that he would sincerely try to reform.

Life in prison continued the brutal existence of the earlier period, but Gary met a woman, Becky, who visited him in prison (she had initially accompanied a friend who was visiting another prisoner), and they planned to marry. She needed to have surgery for an ulcerous condition and died in surgery. After this Gary became even more uncontrolled, and he was scheduled to be put back on prolixin. He arranged with the warden to be transferred to the federal prison in Illinois instead. He left Oregon in January 1975. As he left the prison, he told a friend that he planned to "go get me a couple of Mormons" (Gilmore, 1994, p. 314).

Gary behaved well in the federal prison, and he started writing to a cousin in Utah, Brenda. Gary was eventually paroled to the Utah relatives (Brenda and her husband and Brenda's parents). He was released on April 9, 1976. Years earlier he had said that he would kill a couple of Mormons, and now he had managed to obtain his release to a state where he could accomplish this.

He worked in his uncle's shoe store and met a woman, Nicole, to whom he got engaged. But he started drinking and taking a headache medication which had a powerful effect on his behavior. He got into fights, lost his job, took up stealing, and brutalized Nicole.

One night in July he went driving with Nicole's sister and, with her in the truck, went into a gas station, robbed the 26-year-old attendant, Max Jensen, and shot him in the back of the head, twice. The next night, he walked into a motel in Provo, shot the receptionist, Ben

Bushnell, in the back of the head and stole the cash box. He was recognized and, after he called Brenda for help (he had shot himself in the thumb), was caught in a roadblock.

Asking To Be Executed

At the trial a couple of months later, Gary stared at the judge and jury menacingly, refused to let Nicole testify, and offered his own testimony belligerently. On October 7 he was found guilty and sentenced to death. He told the judge he wanted to be shot rather than hanged. He waived the right to appeal and requested that his execution be carried out. The date was set for Monday November 15. He was apparently seeking a state-sanctioned suicide.

The Utah governor ordered a stay, for which Gary called him a "moral coward." On November 16, both Gary and Nicole attempted suicide by overdosing on sedatives. Bessie and Mikal considered appealing on Gary's behalf. On December 3, the United States Supreme Court ordered a stay of execution but lifted it on December 13. The execution was rescheduled for January 17.

Mikal visited Gary to discuss appeals. Gary told Mikal:

> I killed two men. I don't want to spend the rest of my life in jail. If some fucker gets me set free, then I'm going to go get a gun and kill a few more of those damn lawyers who keep interfering. Then I'll say to you, "See what your meddling accomplish? Are you proud?" (Gilmore, 1994, p. 339)

Frank Jr. felt that:

> Gary had reached the point of no return. He wanted the release of death. . . . He had found the perfect way to beat the system by having them kill him. Then he's out of it. (Gilmore, 1994, p. 341)

Later, Gary told Mikal that, if his sentence was commuted:

> I'd kill myself. (Gilmore, 1994, p. 343)

Gary also told Mikal that at one time he had wanted to murder Mikal. Mikal thought it was because Mikal had managed to escape the Gilmore family, while Gary had not.

Gary Gilmore was executed by shooting on Monday morning, January 17, 1977.

A RECENT CASE

More recent cases of this nature have occurred. For example, John Thanos had a long criminal career, spending most of his 41 years in reform schools and prisons for assault, car theft, rape, and robbery. Thanos had a history of drug and alcohol abuse, and was diagnosed as having an antisocial personality disorder (more commonly known as being a psychopath or sociopath). He tried to kill himself while awaiting trial on his most recent offense, and his friends and relatives said that he had a death wish.

Thanos was raised in a working-class area of Dundalk in eastern Baltimore County. He was the oldest of three children, with two younger sisters, and there were rumors that his father was quite sadistic toward him. He was placed in a juvenile home at the age of 12, sent to a men's prison at 15 where he was raped by the older inmates, and was given a 21-year sentence for rape at age 20 in 1969. He was released in 1986 whereupon he robbed a convenience store and was sent back to prison.

He was then released from prison "by mistake" in April 1990, 18 months too early. He returned home to Joppa, Maryland, and worked for a contractor and a chicken processor. He was charged with indecent exposure on August 25, which was a violation of his parole and could have resulted in his being returned to prison. On August 29, he bought a .22 caliber semiautomatic rifle at a Salisbury sporting goods store and went on a crime spree during which he killed three teenagers. When Thanos was hitchhiking on August 31, 1990, Gregory Taylor aged 18 gave him a ride. Thanos wanted to take his car and money and planned to tie Gregory to a tree but shot him instead. The next day Thanos bought gasoline and paid for the gas with $20 and a gold watch. He went back two days later, on Labor Day, to buy his watch back for $60, as agreed, but the watch was at the home of the girl-friend of the clerk. Thanos then demanded all the money in the cash register and then shot the clerk Billy Winebrenner (aged 16) and his girl-friend Melody Pistorio (aged 14) who was with him that day. Thanos was convicted for these crimes and sentenced to death.

In a telephone conversation with his mother on September 1, 1990, Thanos told her that he had wanted to kill in order to be killed. After his arrest in which he confessed to the murders, he told detectives that he wanted to spare the state the expense of a trial by pleading guilty and being executed. He refused to cooperate with his public defender. After his convictions (in January and March 1992) and sentencing, he showed no remorse, but he also refused further appeals of his death sentence. His mother and sister filed an appeal on his behalf in March 1994, and Thanos wrote to the court complaining about the appeal. He was executed by lethal injection at 1 A.M. on May 17, 1994, the first person executed in Maryland since 1961. He told the execution commander, "Get on with it," and his last words were "Adios. Here it comes now."

The *Baltimore Sun* reported that "Thanos, who had declared himself an outlaw and once said he yearned to die in a blazing gunfight with police, hastened his own execution by refusing to appeal his convictions and opposing attempts by others to spare his life." He is reported to have told police, "I knew I was going to do outrageous things because I wanted the police to be able to come down on me heavy in a shootout so they could put me out of my pain. . . . But it didn't happen that way."

Such cases are not common, and there has been no study of what proportion of offenders sentenced to death are motivated fully or in part by these motivations. Such information would be of great interest.

CHAPTER 9
Murder Followed by Suicide

Some murderers kill themselves immediately after their crime. The frequency of this varies greatly from country to country. Marvin Wolfgang's (1958) study of murder in Philadelphia found that only 4 percent of murderers committed suicide after their murder, whereas in England, where the murder rate is much lower than in America, Donald West (1966) found that 33 percent of murderers committed suicide.

Alan Berman (1979) observed that murder-suicides fell into two types: 1) erotic-aggressive in which an angry lover murders a sexual partner and then commits suicide, and 2) dependent-protective in which a suicidal person kills a dependent in order to prevent them suffering. These latter cases also fall into types. In one, a parent, often a mother, decides to kill herself and worries about how her children will survive after her death. She decides, therefore, to kill them first before killing herself or else she arranges that all will die in the same event. In the other type, an elderly person, perhaps suffering from pain or a terminal illness, kills a spouse who may also be suffering, and then commits suicide.

In Philadelphia, Wolfgang found that the suicide occurred soon after the murder in most cases, and the victim was more likely to be a relative or lover than in other murders. The suicidal murderers were more likely to be male and more often brutal in their killing, perhaps because of greater frustration and anger.

The suicidal murderers were more often white and older, and their victims were younger. The suicidal murders took place more often in the home, and the murder and victim were more often of opposite sex. These suicidal murderers were less often drunk at the time of the murder.

Wolfgang suggested that two possible reasons for these murderers committing suicide after the murder were excessive anger and guilt. However, these murderers were less likely to have prior arrest records and so seem to be more law-abiding and conforming than other murderers. Thus, guilt or the desire to escape punishment seemed to be more likely motives for the suicides.

Wolfgang found that husbands who murdered wives were more likely to commit suicide than wives who killed husbands (19% versus 1%). Wolfgang felt that this difference was a result of the fact that more of the husbands provoked their wives murderous behavior by, for example, beating them, and so their wives felt less guilt after killing their husbands. Wolfgang found that only 9 percent of the wives had played a role in provoking their husbands into killing them versus 60 percent of the husbands.

Theodore Dorpat (1966) studied eight cases of murderers who committed suicide. The suicides in his cases also followed closely upon the murder. The murderer and the victim had an intimate relationship with a great deal of discord, and the murder typically followed a real or threatened separation. Dorpat's murderers were frequently judged to have a psychiatric disorder.

SUICIDE IN THOSE WHO
MURDER COPS

David Lester (1987) noted that from 1974 to 1978, 558 law enforcement officers were murdered in the United States and 729 murderers identified. Of these offenders, 28 (3.4%) committed suicide afterwards, a figure comparable to those who murder other civilians. The suicide rate of those who murder police officers works out to roughly 3,430 per 100,000 per year as compared to a general suicide rate in the United States of about 12.

Lester compared the murderers who committed suicide with those who did not kill themselves. Slightly more of the murder-suicides were white (65% versus 56%), male (100% versus 96%), and aged between 18 to 39 years (66% versus 60%).

All of the murder-suicides used firearms for the murder and 93 percent used guns to commit suicide, including four who used the police officer's gun. The majority of the murder-suicide incidents were not associated with major crimes. Seven involved traffic stops, accidents, or disabled vehicles. Five were family disturbances. In only six cases was the offender involved in an armed robbery or burglary. In addition, one was hijacking an airplane and one was a sniper.

These criminals may have been trying to defend themselves or escape capture, and several seem to have killed themselves while being hunted and when cornered. As arrest became imminent, they killed themselves.

Six of the offenders killed, wounded, or threatened close relatives and, in these cases, the police officer was killed because he was present while the violence was being discharged. A few of the murderers appeared to have grievances against particular police officers since they sought out the home of a police officer or the police station in order to kill the officer.

GIG YOUNG: OSCAR WINNER

An interesting case of murder-suicide is provided by the actor Gig Young who murdered his wife and then committed suicide.[1] Byron Barr was born in St. Cloud, Minnesota, on November 4, 1913, the third of three children and an unplanned baby. His father, stern and distant, ran a pickling and preserving company, his mother was repressed and neurasthenic, and his older brother domineering. Byron was close only to his sister Genevieve and remained so all of his life. In his early years, his mother often took to her room sick and her step-sister, Jessie, came to live with the Barrs to help with the children. Byron grew close to Jessie, but eventually he realized that Jessie liked his older brother, Don, better than she liked him. Thus, both of his female caretakers had rejected him.

Byron developed a number of psychosomatic complaints, including convulsions and a stiff neck, and at elementary school he soon fell behind and was placed with the group of slow learners. His second grade teacher sadistically beat him, and he had to repeat second-grade.

Byron rarely expressed his pain or resentment. He learned to hide behind a smiling countenance, revealing his true feelings only to his sister. His older brother had worked in his father's company successfully, and Byron too was forced to work there after school. There he failed too. The foreman fired him, not realizing he was the boss's son, and his father rehired him but at reduced pay. As a teenager, Byron was attracted by the movies, and he got a job as an usher at the local theater so that he could see the films. He day-dreamt about being an actor.

---

[1] This is based on the biography by George Eells (1991).

At the Technical High School, Byron was a good-looking young man, and he was popular, even getting elected class president. Since his father's business was profitable, Byron had lots of nice clothes and use of the family car, and he developed more self-confidence.

The Depression brought hard times. The father's company folded, and he took a job as a food broker in Washington, D.C., while Byron stayed in St. Cloud to take care of his ailing mother. As he finished his junior year of high school, his father summoned the family to Washington, and so in April 1932, Byron drove his sick and depressed mother to join his father.

Since his father lived far from the high school there, Byron persuaded his parents to let him board near his school. His landlady, Mrs. Harry Kaines, liked him and became his surrogate mother. She was thrilled by his athletic success, and one of her tenants got him a job at the local drug store. When his parents moved to North Carolina, Byron persuaded them to let him stay with Mrs. Kaines. Mrs. Kaines helped get him a job as a ballroom dancing instructor and encouraged him to join the local semi-professional theater group. At this time too, he had the gap in his front teeth closed, and a testicular inflammation forced him to have a vasectomy. Finally, in 1939, he set out for California, hitch-hiking across America.

Arriving in California, Byron got work at a gas station and building scenery at an acting school. He auditioned successfully at the Pasadena Playhouse and acted in many plays. There he met a fellow actress, Sheila Stapler, with whom he fell in love. Sheila was very nurturing and was happy to defer to Byron. They slipped off to Las Vegas in August 1940 to marry.

In 1941, Byron was asked to take a screen test for Warner Brothers,[2] and he was signed for $75 a week. He worked diligently there, but also remained a family man, spending time with Sheila and working on his house.

When America entered the war in 1941, the movie studios lost many male actors, and Warner Brothers persuaded Byron not to enlist. They upgraded the roles given to Byron, and he took as his name the role he played in *The Gay Sisters,* Gig Young. His next film was *Old Acquaintance* with Bette Davis, and Gig and Bette had an affair, a portent that Gig was most likely not going to be a stable husband.

Gig finally had to enlist, joining the Coast Guard in 1943, but Sheila moved to be with him until he was shipped off to sea as a

---

[2] His father sent him funds so that he could join the Screen Actors Guild.

pharmacist's mate in late 1944, just after his mother died. He got malaria soon afterwards and was released on July 4, 1945. Warner Brothers threw a welcome back party for him and several other returning actors, and Gig hoped that his fortunes would improve. However, Warner Brothers gave him second-string and unflattering roles in many of their run-of-the-mill movies, and the momentum of his career slowed.

He grew closer to Sophie Rosenstein, a drama coach for the studio (the two couples socialized a lot together), and Gig and Sophie fell in love. Sophie worked hard to encourage Gig and to help him land better roles. She urged him to act on the stage in order to expand his horizons, but in the summer of 1947, while he was appearing in *Biography* at the La Jolla Playhouse, Warner Brothers dropped his option. His brother Don died, in September 1949, of tubercular meningitis and, although he had always resented his brother, Gig was depressed by this loss. His marriage to Sheila deteriorated, and, as his drinking increased, Gig took to breaking the furniture during their rows. They separated after Christmas 1948 and divorced in 1949. Gig persuaded Sophie to divorce her husband, and they married on January 1, 1951.

Working as an independent, Gig let his agent sign him up for mediocre roles and, after getting and breaking a contract with Columbia, he hardly worked in 1949 and 1950. He freelanced a few roles in 1951, but then signed with the Louis Shurr Agency. He obtained a good part and turned in a good performance in *Come Fill The Cup* for which he was nominated as best supporting actor in 1952. But then he signed with MGM who put him in mediocre films, and his career fizzled again.

He failed to insist on better roles, and Sophie could not help him since she was diagnosed with cervical cancer just three months after their marriage. Gig held the knowledge from Sophie and spent much of his energy taking care of her. By October 1952, she spent most of her time in bed, and Gig stayed home with her. She had to be hospitalized in October 1952, and she died on November 10. Gig was devastated and seriously depressed. He drank heavily and took Miltown to help him sleep. When his contract with MGM expired, Gig decided to go to New York to act on the stage. He got his first part in *Oh Men! Oh Women!* in 1953 and received great reviews. He also began to recover from his bereavement, and had two affairs. First there was Sherry Britton, a big-time stripper, to whom Gig proposed marriage. She refused.[3] Elaine Stritch was acting in a show in a neighboring theater

---

[3] She reported that Gig was unable to have an orgasm for months at a time.

and met Gig at a party she gave. He stayed overnight to help her wash dishes and slept in a separate bed. The virgin Elaine was impressed, and they began dating. Soon she fell in love with him, and Gig tried to have his first marriage annulled and planned to convert to Roman Catholicism in order to marry her. After they went back to Hollywood where Gig had a role in a movie, the church found out that he had been baptized as a Methodist, and so an annulment was impossible. Their relationship broke up soon after.

For a while, Gig shuttled back and forth between New York and Hollywood, but he found few good roles and took any that were offered. He met Elizabeth Montgomery, and they married in December 1956. Gig had his vasectomy reversed so they could have children. Gig had a good role in *Teacher's Pet* which got him a second Oscar nomination. This led to several offers, and Gig and Liz moved to the West Coast. Gig was still drinking heavily, but Liz seemed to be able to match him in this.

Returning to the East Coast for *Under The Yum Yum Tree,* Gig began to show signs of what later became a severe problem, his inability to master the lines for a play. As his marriage with Liz deteriorated, Gig found a new mother-figure, Doris Rich, a character actress in her mid-sixties, a relationship which made Liz feel insecure. Gig next had a liaison with Sophia Loren during the filming of *Five Miles To Midnight* in 1962; yet he was worried about Liz having affairs! Liz obtained a Mexican divorce in March 1963.

Gig drowned his sorrows in alcohol, but he soon met Elaine Whitman who was, at the time, selling real estate. Soon after their affair began, Elaine discovered she was pregnant, and Gig, overjoyed, married her, though friends thought it was a terrible match. Elaine was 28, Gig 49. Elaine and Gig had a daughter, Jennifer, in April 1964. Elaine tried domesticity, while Gig tried AA, dieted, and acquired toupees for his receding hairline. His failing career soon brought financial worries. He starred in a television series for a year, *The Rogues,* but it was canceled. He was in a successful touring company of *The Music Man,* but he had to sell his luxurious house and move into a smaller place.

Gig's paranoia now focussed on Elaine, and he tapped his own telephone line so as to record her conversations. Gig persuaded Elaine to go into counseling with him, but he chose an unqualified therapist. Elaine refused to continue, and Gig went to Vancouver for a course of LSD therapy. Their arguments about Gig's drinking continued and Elaine divorced Gig in July 1967.

Gig was now getting almost no offers for films, and appeared only in touring companies and occasionally in New York City. An affair there with a young actress was ruined by his drinking and his impotence and, although she would have married him, Gig refused to consider it. At this nadir in his life, he was recommended for the role of Rockie Gravo in *They Shoot Horses, Don't They?* and he won an Oscar for best supporting actor in 1970 for his performance.

And then his career plummeted again! Elaine sued him in court for more alimony and child support, and Gig tried to deny paternity for Jennifer. He lost in court after five years of legal battles which created great animosity between them, and Gig never saw Jennifer again. Furthermore, public opinion turned against him. Then, in his touring company for *Harvey,* there was great conflict between Gig and other actors and, though the production was a success, Gig acquired a reputation for being difficult. The stress of this experience led to a severe neurodermatitis on his face.

Next, Gig was hired for a film, *Blazing Saddles,* but he had problems learning the lines, and his anxiety caused him to collapse on the set. He was fired. His reputation for being unreliable grew. Luckily though, he found another supporter, Harriette Vine Douglas, a woman in her fifties, who became his friend, confidante, and lover. She protected him in every way she could, and he often hid out with her for months.

He tried plastic surgery for his aging face, but the surgeon botched the operation, and Gig required remedial surgery. His teeth bothered him so that, on tour with *On A Clear Day You Can See Forever,* he could hardly eat. After his weight dropped from 185 to 145, he had all of his teeth recapped. In 1972, he developed numbness in his feet and was treated for circulatory problems and had his gallbladder removed. After this, he stayed with Harriette for almost a year.

In 1974 and 1975 he appeared in five movies. He went on the wagon, relying more heavily on Valium and Placidyl, and he made a television movie which became a series. He had problems learning the lines and hired a good psychologist who helped him. But after the series, when the psychologist tried to get Gig to deal with his underlying and chronic problems (his alcoholism, sexual impotence, and paranoia), Gig quit therapy. Gig had his teeth redone and had plastic surgery on his chin and eyelids.

Back in New York, he was fired from Arthur Miller's *The Archbishop's Ceiling* because he could not remember his lines, despite help from his voice-coach there, Bert Knapp, who had managed also to become Gig's therapist although unqualified for such a role. In 1977 Gig went to Hong Kong to make a kung fu film (his last film) and met Kim Schmidt.

Kim was the 30-year-old script girl for the film, and they soon became involved. Their relationship was volatile, and Kim desperately tried to get Gig to stop drinking. Gig returned to New York alone, but the relationship improved by telephone, and Kim joined him in New York in October 1977.

He signed up to perform in a college production of *Long Day's Journey Into Night* at the University of Memphis, where his memorization problems led to the first performance ending 45 minutes early as Gig forget large chunks of his lines. Back in New York, Gig and Kim quarreled, made up, split, and got back together again. Gig proposed marriage, but Kim resisted. In May, Gig appeared drunk on stage when introducing a friend's concert performance, and his voice-coach/psychotherapist broke his relationship with Gig. In June 1978, Gig and Kim went to Edmonton where Gig was to perform in *Nobody Loves An Albatross*. Gig had fantasies of taking the show on tour, but friends who came to advise him on it thought the production was terrible.

Back in New York, Gig and Kim bought an apartment and, on September 27, 1978, finally married. Money was scarce because of their heavy spending and the expense of fixing up the apartment.

Perhaps it was the fears of aging and sickness, perhaps his sexual impotence or arguments over money, perhaps it was a fight over the will (with Kim wanting all the inheritance and Gig wanting to split it between Kim and his sister), or perhaps his withdrawal from alcohol and drugs led to an acute psychosis? He telephoned Harriette on October 18 to beg her to come to New York and take him back to Hollywood. She refused.

On October 19, 1978, Gig shot Kim in the back of the head and then shot himself in the head. After the deaths, no barbiturates or alcohol were found in Gig's system. The apartment had two bottles of wine, seven tablets of Oxazepam, and several bottles of vitamins.

Gig Young was a man whose life disintegrated slowly, interspersed with occasional successes and critical turning points. From a difficult childhood, filled with rejection, he built a career, but he lacked the skills to manage it well. As he progressed from relationship to relationship and from performance to performance, his alcohol abuse worsened, his distrust of others and paranoia worsened, and his violent behavior escalated. The eventual end of his life was hardly predictable. Murder-suicide is rare, but Gig's decline was inevitable, perhaps into bankruptcy and alcoholism.

But there were also critical turning points. What if Sophie, his second wife, had not died of cancer? He loved her, and she was good for him and his career. What if he had not quit the qualified psychotherapist he had found but stayed to work through his problems? What if?

Suicide-by-Cop:
A Look at the Issues

CHAPTER 10

Suicide-By-Cop and African Americans

African Americans have relatively low suicide rates in the United States. For example, in 1990, David Lester (1998a) reported that the suicide rate for white males was 22.0 per 100,000 per year and for black males 12.0. The suicide rate for white females was 5.3 and for black females 2.3.

Some commentators on this difference have noted that some black suicides may be disguised, and one of the ways of disguising a suicide is to have someone else kill you, including a police officer. Marvin Wolfgang (1958), in his study of victim-precipitated homicide discussed in Chapter 7, did find that this behavior was more common among African Americans than among whites. Perhaps suicide-by-cop is also more common among African Americans than among whites? However, as we have seen in chapter 2, the vast majority of perpetrators of suicide-by-cop incidents are white.

Jewell Gibbs (1988) suggested that the aggressive and anti-authority behavior of the Black Panthers in the 1960s and 1970s fitted the pattern of suicide-by-cop, for several of them were killed in gun battles with the police. Hugh Pearson (1994) has documented the history of the Black Panthers, with examples of Huey Newton brandishing a gun in front of Oakland police officers while threatening them, even to the point of loading it in their presence. In one confrontation, Bobby Hutton was shot by police after a half-hour gun battle with police in West Oakland in which two officers were wounded. Although Hutton and others eventually surrendered to the police, Hutton stumbled while walking and dropped his arms, whereupon the police shot and killed him.

It should be noted, however, that some commentators disagree with this interpretation that suicide was appealing to the Black Panthers.

Charles and Betty Valentine (1972) noted that the original name for the group was "Black Panther Party for Self-Defense," and self-defense is the opposite of self-destruction. The Black Panthers established and maintained many community services and programs, but it was also committed to revolutionary change. Indeed, the party argued that to accept white oppression was a form of collective suicide. Revolutionary action was seen as opposing this collective suicide. If African Americans did nothing, that would be self-murder. Working for revolutionary change might result in some members of the party being killed, but self-destruction was clearly not the *goal* of the party.

Frank Donner (1990) has also documented the actions of the police in America in protecting the economic and political interests of the capitalist system, activities which included repressive tactics such as dragnet and pretext arrests, the use of force to disperse gatherings, indiscriminate clubbings, and support for vigilante offensives. The police infiltrated organizations, including the Black Panthers, and raided these organizations in a confrontational manner in order to maximize the intimidation. Even though those persecuted by the police sometimes won in court, as did members of the Black Panthers in New York in May 1971, the time spent in jail and in court fights often led to the dismemberment of the organization.

Members of the Symbionese Liberation Army died in a fire after a gun battle with the police, as did the members of MOVE in Philadelphia in 1986, and these incidents might be viewed as motivated by suicidal desires, at least in part. Let us look at one of these incidents, the confrontations between MOVE and the Philadelphia Police Department, in some detail.

THE MOVE CONFRONTATIONS

Michael and Randi Boyette (1989) have described the two confrontations between MOVE members and the Philadelphia police which eventually resulted in the deaths of eleven members.

John Africa, the leader of the group, was born as Vincent Leaphart in 1931 in Philadelphia. He left school early, was arrested for armed robbery and car theft, but then joined the army and served in Korea. After he returned to Philadelphia, his odd behavior became more noticeable. He used candles rather than electricity, furnished his house with junk he took from trash, hated to kill any creature (even insects), and walked dogs for a living. After a brief marriage ended in divorce, Vincent began to develop a philosophy of living and formed the Christian Movement for Life, known simply as MOVE. He bought a house in Powelton Village on North 33rd Street in Philadelphia and began to recruit followers. His commune ate raw food, even meat, and did not use furniture or modern conveniences such as electricity, gas, or running water.[1] Their excrement was simply thrown into the yard. At that time, Vincent predicted that there would be a conflagration, a time when the adults and children would die.

They began to protest around Philadelphia. For example, they wanted the zoo to set the animals free, and they protested against Jane Fonda, Dick Gregory, Jesse Jackson, and Mike Douglas. In 1973, the police logged 10 demonstrations with no arrests; in 1975 there were 38 demonstrations with 142 arrests.

Eventually neighbors protested. The MOVE members began to acquire guns and bombs, the confrontations with the police escalated, and the city decided it had to act. The Mayor, Frank Rizzo, gave the order on August 8, 1978. The police sealed off the block and moved in a bulldozer to demolish the MOVE houses. Eventually a gun battle ensued. The MOVE members shot one police officer, James Ramp, and five other police officers and firemen were wounded by gunshots. Tear gas was used, and the MOVE members fled the house, whereupon most were arrested. Eleven were convicted for the murder of Officer Ramp.

The group dispersed, but in the 1980s began to drift back into Philadelphia. Vincent acquired a house in the 62nd hundred block of Osage Avenue, and the same situation developed as before. The new mayor, Wilson Goode, tried to ignore the problem, but eventually he too decided he had to act, and on May 13, 1985, the police tried to evict and arrest the MOVE members. This time the police decided to drop a bomb on the roof to dislodge a bunker that the group had erected on the top of their row home. The house caught fire, and the authorities decided to let the house burn. Eventually the whole block of houses caught fire, and 61 houses were destroyed. Six adults, including Vincent, and five children died in the MOVE house in the fire.

Vincent had provoked the conflagration that he had predicted.

---

[1] They had pets which they fed, and they also fed the rats!

CHAPTER 11

Legal Issues in Suicide-by-Cop

Suicide-by-cop raises several legal issues and can cause problems for law enforcement agencies. The relatives of the perpetrator of a suicide-by-cop incident can sue the law enforcement agency for unjustifiably killing the suspect, and, if he survives, so can the perpetrator. Since law enforcement agencies do kill suspects justifiably on some occasions and unjustifiably on other occasions, it is important that psychological and law enforcement experts establish clear criteria for classifying accurately suicide-by-cop incidents so that legal challenges can be withstood.[1]

In *Saunders v. City of Santa Rosa, et al.* (Doc. #216194. Sup. Ca., 1998), Robert Homant and his colleagues (2000) noted that Saunders, in a suicide-by-cop situation, was shot and killed by police, after which it was found that he was unarmed. His family sued the city, and the lawsuit was settled by summary judgment for the defense in December 1998. Saunders had raised his hands when commanded to do so by police officers, but he then lowered his hands to his waist, suggesting to the police officers (but not to all bystanders) that he was going to draw a weapon.

Homant pointed out that the law requires that a hypothetical, reasonable police officer would view the situation as threatening before he fires his weapon, and in law this is called an *objective* test. Homant noted that a psychologist would view this as a *perpetratorive* test because it is based on the *perceived* threat and not on the *actual* danger involved. Saunders was perceived as a threat, but he did not possess a gun and so was not an actual threat.

[1] More cases relevant to suicide-by-cop have been reviewed by Robert Miller (2001).

In their study, Homant and his colleagues collected 123 published accounts of suicide-by-cop incidents. In 6.5 percent of these incidents, one or more people were killed by the perpetrator, in 6.5 percent one or more people were wounded by the perpetrator, in 43.1 percent police or bystanders were directly threatened by the perpetrator, in 22.0 percent the police were indirectly threatened or attacked by a makeshift or less-dangerous weapon, in 9.8 percent the perpetrator possessed an empty or inoperable firearm, and in 12.2 percent the perpetrator used a prop or bluffed having a firearm. The first four categories involved real danger—someone was already or could have been seriously hurt.

The last two categories appeared to have posed real danger, but in fact did not. Homant scored each of the 123 incidents for whether they involved real danger or not. However, category number 4 above (the police were indirectly threatened or attack by a makeshift or less dangerous weapon) covers incidents that are perceived by police officers as dangerous, but in fact are not. Perpetrators possessing empty or inoperable weapons (category 5) or bluffing having a firearm (category 6) are in fact not dangerous, but the police officers have no way of knowing this at the time. Homant scored all 123 incidents for "perceived danger," that is, whether they were category 4 incidents (the police were indirectly threatened or attack by a makeshift or less dangerous weapon) or not.

For all 123 incidents, the association between the real danger score and the perceived danger score was positive but very weak. Furthermore, real danger did not predict whether the perpetrator died, whereas perceived danger did.

In those incidents where the perpetrator had an empty or inoperable gun or bluffed having a gun (categories 5 and 6), he was more likely to be killed than in the other incidents (89% of the time versus 68% of the time). Thus, Homant concluded that police officers are unable to distinguish actual threats from bluffs.

The age and sex of the perpetrator were unrelated to real danger, perceived danger, or a fatal outcome. Those perpetrators who planned the suicide-by-cop incident created incidents that were less dangerous to others (that is, real danger) but more lethal to the self. Incidents whose perpetrators had personal psychopathology did not differ in real or perceived dangerousness, but the perpetrators were more likely to end up dead. The presence of others in the suicide-by-cop increased the real danger and the perceived danger and increased the likelihood of a fatal outcome.

Homant and his colleagues found a federal appellate case (*Palmquist v. Selvis 111F 3d 1332, 7th Circuit 1997*) which noted that identification of an incident as a suicide-by-cop can be relevant in three ways in a wrongful death lawsuit: 1) if police officers are aware of the perpetrator's suicidal motivation, this might have a bearing on their tactics and level of force; 2) if there is a dispute about facts, such as the perpetrator's movements, suicidal motivation might have probative value (that is, value as evidence); and/or 3) the extent of the perpetrator's suicidal motivation might have relevance to the amount of damages, if any.

In 1998, the United States Supreme Court held that cities can be sued for inadequate police training that leads to death or injury, even in situations where suicidal individuals threaten police officers with weapons. Thus, it is important that police departments provide adequate training for their officers in the use of deadly force and that they continually update this training with in-service sessions for experienced officers.

GUIDELINES FOR ESTABLISHING AN INCIDENT AS SUICIDE-BY-COP

Establishing that the perpetrator of a police shooting intended that the police shoot him requires the exploration of several factors.

Stressors

Suicides are found to have experienced more life stress than nonsuicidal people, and the stress has increased further in the period leading up to the suicide. Therefore, it is important to find out if the perpetrator was under severe stress. In a case in which one of us was a consultant, the perpetrator was wanted by the police as a suspect in a case of homicide. He had recently broken-up with his girl-friend, and the girl-friend had obtained a restraining order to prevent him contacting her or their daughter. The perpetrator was fearful of going to prison. All the stressors had been chronic, that is, lasting for six or more months.

Profile

As we saw in Chapter 2, we have some idea of what the typical suicide-by-cop perpetrator is like. In the case above, the perpetrator had some of these characteristics.

1. He was of low socio-eoconomic status.
2. He had a criminal history.

In addition, other important background characteristics include:

3. a psychiatric disorder (and prior psychiatric treatment),
4. a history of drug or alcohol abuse,
5. symptoms of depression and talk of suicide. The perpetrator may give subtle clues to possible suicidal intent by giving away personal possession or making final arrangements (such as a will). At autopsy, there may be drugs and/or alcohol in the perpetrator's system, a common occurrence in suicides which makes it easier perhaps for them to carry out their suicidal intentions.

The event itself also provides clues as to whether the situation was one of suicide-by-cop. In suicide-by-cop situations:

1. The incident is initiated by the perpetrator or by a third party, not by the police. The perpetrator may approach the police or cause an action that will lead others to call the police.
2. The precipitating event ensures a police presence. Since the perpetrator wishes to die at the hands of the police, he will create an incident that is designed to bring the police to him.
3. The perpetrator forces the confrontation. Instead of surrendering, the perpetrator will take actions that escalate the incident, such as taking an aggressive stance.
4. The perpetrator initiates the aggressive action, such as openly displaying a weapon, in order to heighten the police officers' fear level.
5. There is a weapon present which increases the likelihood that the police will fire at the suspect. However, on some occasions, the perpetrator acts in such a way that the police assume he has a weapon even though he does not.
6. The perpetrator threatens the police officers with the weapon. Since the perpetrator needs the police to kill him, he places the officers in fear of their lives.
7. The perpetrator refuses to drop the weapon when the police demand that he do so. If he were to drop the weapon, this would de-escalate the situation and interrupt the suicidal process.
8. The perpetrator threatens the police officers by body language, facial contortions, or words. He may approach or appear to advance toward the police officers, reinforcing the assumption that he is aggressive and dangerous, thereby escalating the incident.
9. Even if the police officers retreat, this does not defuse the situation. Typically, the police in these situations retreat out of fear for their lives, not simply for cover or concealment. Police officers state that, in these situations, they knew someone was going to die.

10. If there is only one officer present, he will not be harmed, for he is to be the agent of death. If there are civilians or additional officers present, the perpetrator may attempt to harm them or actually harm them in order to escalate the incident.

In 23 cases we examined, the percentage of incidents in which some of the above criteria were met was as follows:

recent stressors	65%
mental illness/chronic physical illness	61%
drug/alcohol abuse	78%
low socioeconomic background	78%
prior suicidal behavior	39%
criminal history	65%
incident not initiated by police	96%
precipitating event to ensure police presence	100%
perpetrator forces confrontation	96%
perpetrator initiated aggressive action	100%
presence of a deadly weapon	100%
officer threatened with weapon	83%
perpetrator advances toward police	74%
perpetrator refuses to drop weapon	100%
perpetrator threatens civilian or officer	65%
officer or civilian injured	35%
retreat by officers	83%

Remember, in the above cases, sometimes the information on the perpetrators' personal characteristics or recent stressors was not always discovered, and not all reports of the incidents recorded all of the necessary information on the incident.

CHAPTER 12
Hostage Negotiations

Negotiating with those involved in hostage or barricade incidents is a comparatively recent strategy developed by law enforcement agencies. Michael McMains and Wayman Mullins (1996) noted that, prior to the 1970s, an assault was the most common tactic used in these situations, as illustrated at the Olympic Games in Munich in 1972 when a group of Arabs invaded the Israeli compound at the games and took Israeli athletes as hostages. In the assault at the airport, police killed 10 Arabs, and 11 Israelis and lost one police officer. Beginning in the 1970s, law enforcement agencies realized that some situations could be resolved by negotiations, and guidelines gradually evolved for handling such situations.

McMains and Mullins observed that not every situation is negotiable. A negotiable incident has eight characteristics. First, the hostage-taker has to want to live, for without this desire on the part of the perpetrator, the negotiator has little with which to bargain. Second, the authorities have to threaten to use force, and this threat must be a credible one so that the perpetrator will believe it. Third, the hostage taker must make demands; the demands make negotiation possible and buy time for the negotiators.

Fourth, the negotiator must be perceived by the perpetrator as both a person who can hurt him and who is also willing to help him. Fifth, there must be sufficient time for the negotiator to develop a relationship with the perpetrator and for the negotiations to proceed. Sixth, there must be a channel of communication between the negotiator and the perpetrator, and this involves technical equipment (such as a telephone line) and skills on the part of the negotiator. Seventh, the locale needs to be contained to prevent others from intruding into the situation. This involves not only the physical locale, but also the channel of communication (that is, the perpetrator's telephone lines and other means of communication with others must be isolated). Finally, if there is more than one hostage-taker, the negotiator must deal with the one who makes the decisions.

Without these eight conditions, negotiation becomes difficult. In situations in which there are no hostages or where the perpetrator makes no demands, negotiation is less likely to defuse the situation, and the police may have to resort to assault, accurate sniper fire, or the use of chemical agents (such as tear gas).

THE PRINCIPLES OF NEGOTIATION

Situations Which May Involve Negotiation

Once a negotiation team has been established by a police department, the team members may be involved in a wide variety of situations, including people who barricade themselves in their homes, those contemplating suicide (such as people who have climbed onto a building roof or ledge in order to jump to their deaths), domestic disputes, prison riots, the apprehension of mentally-disturbed people, serving warrants to dangerous felons, stalking incidents, and debriefing those involved in violent crisis incidents (such as for those who have shot a suspect or been involved in search-and-rescue operations with mass casualties).

Crisis Intervention

Perpetrators are often in a crisis state, and sometimes the negotiation team has to engage in crisis intervention with the perpetrator. Crisis intervention in general involves three stages. First, the crisis intervener uses active listening. In active listening, which is based on person-centered psychotherapy devised by Carl Rogers, the counselor tries to get the client to discuss what has happened to them, how they feel about it, and their thoughts about it. The counselor may simply repeat back to the client what he or she has just said, the counselor may paraphrase what the client has said, or the counselor may probe the client's thoughts and feelings by asking questions. The goal is simply to try to understand the client's psychological state.

The second stage is to assess the client's resources, psychological and interpersonal. What strengths do they have and to whom could they turn for help. Finally, the counselor and client must come up with solutions, and the best solutions are the ones that the client suggests, for then the client is much more likely to follow through with the suggestion. McMains and Mullins suggested that brainstorming is good here; that is, throwing out all kinds of possible solutions and then choosing what seems to be the best one. In the context of barricade situations, the brainstorming can also take place between the negotiator and his or her colleagues during time-outs from talking with the perpetrator of the incident.

Handling Demands

Often perpetrators will make demands. McMains and Mullins distinguished between those demands which are negotiable and those which are not. In general, perpetrators should never be promised or given weapons or illegal drugs, and negotiators should never agree to release prisoners or exchange hostages. Negotiators should never ask the perpetrator for his demands but rather wait for the perpetrator to make demands. The negotiator should never offer anything, give anything not specifically requested, and give no more than is absolutely necessary. Finally, the negotiator should never give anything without getting something in return, a hostage if possible, but an agreement for the perpetrator to remain calm and keep talking may be a reasonable trade in some situations.

McMains and Mullins suggest that concessions may include food, cigarettes (and, separately, matches), soft drinks, alcohol, and media coverage. Transportation and money can be negotiated, but negotiators should endeavor not to deliver on these trades if possible. Court decisions have established that agreements made by negotiators during such negotiations are not legally binding since they were made under duress.

McMains and Mullins observed that negotiators should resist any desire to push for a quick resolution to the negotiations, even if their supervisors urge them to do so. It is important to use the negotiations to buy time. Over time, the basic physiological needs of the perpetrator will grow, and the negotiator can use the food and drink to gain the trust of the perpetrator and reduce his anxiety. McMains and Mullins suggest working through the five basic needs of people suggested by Abraham Maslow—physiological, safety and security, belonging, esteem, and self-actualization. After satisfying the perpetrator's physiological needs, with enough time the negotiator can discuss how to satisfy the safety needs of the perpetrator (such as what will happen to him after the incident is resolved), the belonging needs (especially if the negotiator can build up a personal relationship with the perpetrator), esteem needs (by letting the perpetrator know that others care about him, for example), and self-actualization needs (by discussing the perpetrator's future potential, as a husband or father, worker, or even through his hobbies). All of this requires time.

Time also decreases the emotionality of the perpetrator and increases his rationality. If he was drunk, the passage of time results in a more sober person and allows the adrenaline from the initial stressful events to dissipate.

Time also permits the negotiator's team to gather information about the perpetrator, for the police response to be planned, for hostages to escape, and, if a tactical assault is an option, for the assault to be prepared. Sometimes, the perpetrator simply quits after time has passed.

On the other hand, time can increase the fatigue of the perpetrator and the negotiator, and both may behave irrationally as a result.

The Stockholm Syndrome

In 1973, two robbers held up a bank and took four employees hostage. After the 130-hour siege ended, with no casualties, the hostages showed great sympathy toward the robbers and refused to testify against them, and one later became engaged to one of the robbers.

McMains and Mullins observed that negotiators should help this so-called Stockholm syndrome develop. It is useful if the perpetrator bonds with the hostages, for then he will be much less likely to harm them. The perpetrator should be encouraged to find out the hostages' names and to use them, and to find out if the hostages have any illnesses or injuries which need medical attention.

The needs of the hostages should be considered, as well as those of the perpetrator, as the negotiations proceed. For example, everyone should be provided with food if this is one of the demands which is negotiated. The negotiator should not refer to the hostages as "hostages" but rather as "people" or by their names. Time also will develop a relationship between the perpetrator and the hostages. If the perpetrator dehumanizes the hostages (for example, by calling them by demeaning labels), the negotiator can insist on the perpetrator using the hostages' real names in return for satisfying some of the perpetrator's demands.

Roles

The negotiator can assume several roles during the negotiations. He can be a concerned, caring and interested listener, a reasonable problem-solver, someone who commiserates with the perpetrator ("Buddy/Fellow-Traveler"), dumb but trying (in the way that Columbo is in the television series of that name), or a firm, accepting-directing non-judgmental and helpful person. In the course of a long negotiation, the negotiator may have to switch from one of these roles to another, depending on how the situation is developing. Argument and power-plays, however, typically do not work well and tend to alienate the perpetrator.

There are many sets of guidelines for negotiating, which can come from such diverse fields as psychotherapy, management (such as William Ury's book *Getting Past No*), and social psychology (such as Robert Cialdini's *Influence*).

Negotiating A Prison Riot

Fuselier, Van Zandt, and Lancely (1989) discussed the principles guiding the negotiations in two prison hostage situations in November 1987. In the Oakdale, Louisiana, Correctional Facility and in the United States Penitentiary in Atlanta, Georgia, groups of Cuban refugees took over the prisons and held staff members as hostages.

Teams of negotiators were formed at both facilities involving FBI personnel and staff from the Bureau of Prisons which included Spanish-speaking negotiators. Several tactics were utilized.

1. It was important to identify which of the inmates were the leaders. Talking to others did not lead to much progress, but it was difficult for the first few days to identify which of the inmates were leaders and had the ability to influence the other inmates.

2. The negotiators found that it was important to allow time to pass and not to offer too much too soon. Giving in to the demands of the inmates immediately did not allow them to express their anger and frustration at the government. The situation had to "mature" to allow the inmates to ventilate their feelings.

3. The negotiators devised guidelines to measure their progress, including: i) no one injured or killed since the negotiations began; ii) a decrease in the frequency of threats of violence; iii) the inmate's voice is lower, the rate of speech slower, he talks for longer periods of time and he talks about more personal things; iv) hostages have been released; and v) deadlines have passed.

4. It is necessary to avoid tricks and dishonesty so that the inmates build up trust with the negotiators. In particular, if tactical assaults were going to be initiated by the law enforcement officials, the negotiators had to be told in advance so that they could help the inmates prepare for the assaults.

5. Initially, the negotiators in these prisons riots used English-speaking negotiators so that the negotiating sessions were less

emotional and more rational. This also made the negotiations under-standable to all involved. However, conducting the negotiations in English prevented the inmates from ventilating. Eventually, in both prisons, Spanish-speaking negotiators were used when the Cubans asked for particular Spanish-speaking people by name.

6. All negotiations were tape-recorded. This enabled everyone involved to listen to what had transpired, and it also permitted the situations to be used as learning experiences for the future.

7. The use of non-police negotiators did not prove to be very useful. Attorneys, media representatives, and Cuban exiles seemed to produce more ventilation but little progress. On the other hand, Bureau of Prison mental health and correctional personnel greatly assisted in the negotiations. They had experience from previous prison hostage situations, understood the situation of the inmates better, and personally knew some of the inmates.

8. The surrender ritual was important and required great planning so that it would satisfy the inmates. The inmates had a need to orchestrate this ritual, and the negotiators allowed this. For example, at the Oakdale facility a document was signed in the presence of witnesses and the media, and after this the inmates piled their weapons in open view and formed a gauntlet through which the hostages passed.

The particular inmates in these prison situations also presented cultural and behavioral problems. For example, the negotiators had to learn to disregard some of the rhetoric used by the inmates, such as their threats of "rivers of blood." Several inmates eventually told the negotiators that this was "just the way we talk."

The negotiators also learned that these particular inmates did not like to make trades. Instead, they preferred unilateral gestures, after which the other side would respond. After learning this, when the inmates released some hostages the negotiators gave them their mail and turned on the water supply without any of this being neogtiated.

SUICIDE-BY-COP

Although all hostage/barricade incidents have the potential to be complex and deadly, by far the most risky is that involving suicide-by-cop. When an individual decides that life is no longer worth living and that it is time to end it all, most individuals will take their life by their own hand. A few will kill a loved-one or someone else prior to taking their own life. In suicide-by-cop, it seems that the individuals do not have the internal resources needed to kill themselves, and so they create an incident that will force the police to become the weapon of death.

Do police officers respond to a hostage/barricade incident that appears to be a suicide-by-cop situation differently from the way they respond to others? The answer is yes for a variety of reasons.

Most negotiators who have been in the business for any length of time begin to develop a "feel" for the threats that the perpetrator makes toward the victims he has taken hostage. During the first hour or two, the perpetrator will make repeated threats concerning the hostages, even to the point of parading them in front of windows or pointing weapons at them. As the negotiations proceed and the perpetrator becomes the center of attention, the frequency of threats to the hostages diminishes. The negotiator may be able to manipulate the hostage-taker so that there comes a point in time when the life and safety of the hostage-taker is intertwined with that of the hostages. Negotiators are trained to gain control of the incident and then begin to de-escalate the incident until such times as they can obtain a negotiated settlement.

In those incidents where the intent of the perpetrator is to die at the hands of the police, the normal hostage/barricade training is not always applicable. As we have noted above, negotiators are trained to get control of the situation and de-escalate it but, in suicide-by-cop situations, the perpetrator cannot allow this to occur. He maintains control of the situation and continually escalates the incident. Therefore, the perpetrator will not only threaten the hostages but, if the police fail to react to these threats, he will escalate the threats. If the perpetrator has more than one hostage, the likelihood of a hostage being seriously injured or killed increases. Each move that the police make to de-escalate the situation will be countered with a move that heightens the level of tension.

Thus, when the police first suspect that they are dealing with a potential suicide-by-cop situation, they must also begin to plan for an eventual tactical action or assault by the counter-sniper team to end the situation.

If there is time, it is important before negotiations commence to gather as much information about the perpetrator as possible. Police officers can be sent to interview family members, friends, neighbors, and colleagues to obtain information, especially related to prior criminal and medical/psychiatric problems. If the perpetrator has been in an institution (jail, prison, or psychiatric hospital), the records should be obtained to get some feel for his background.

Guidelines For Police

Gary Noesner and John Dolan (1992) noted that the first police officers who respond to a suicide-by-cop incident should take as little action as possible until additional resources have been summoned and have arrived on the scene. The responding officers should hold their position, try to evacuate innocent bystanders, and take action only to save lives.

At the most, they can try to engage the perpetrator in conversation, enabling the perpetrator to ventilate his emotions and regain some self-control. For this, the training of police officers should involve verbal and communication skills, skills which would help officers, not only in suicide-by-cop incidents but in all interactions with civilians.

Clinton Van Zandt (undated) has suggested that, when a situation is identified as a possible suicide-by-cop, the police response should be low-key and non-dramatic. Using lights and sirens for the police cars may serve to escalate the situation, as will the arrival and presence of the media. The more dramatic the scene becomes, the more likely the perpetrator may feel compelled to go through with his perceived role in the drama.

Time is crucial. The more time elapses, the better able the police will be to appraise the sitatuation, contain the crisis and defuse it, and plan tactics. The police must make the safety of any hostages and control of the situation priorities.

Michael McMains and Wayman Mullins (1996) have published checklists for determining whether a barricaded person is a potential suicide-by-cop which involved assessing how suicidal the person is and how aggressive he is. The suicidal checklist included such factors as:

> previous suicide attempts
> lethality of previous attempts
> having a current suicide plan
> alcohol/drug use
> past psychiatric history
> current depression

The aggression checklist included such factors as:

> age (17-25)
> race (black)
> sex (male)
> substance abuse
> low intelligence
> prior arrests for violent offences
> cruelty to animals
> abused as a child
> frequent residential moves
> unemployed or frequent job changes

In suicide-by-cop-situations, the perpetrator may refuse to negotiate with the police, offer to surrender in person to the police officer in charge, demand that they kill him, or set a deadline for them to kill him. He may have recently murdered a significant person in his life or received notification that he has a fatal disease. He may indicate that he has made plans for his death or recently given away or disposed of his property or money. He may present no demands that involve his escape or freedom or give the negotiators a verbal will. He may have a history of assaultive behavior and recent traumatic losses and express feelings of depression and hopelessness.

CHAPTER 13
Helping the Police Officer

Suicide-by-cop incidents have many repercussions. They can worsen police-community relations if the residents think that the police shooting was unnecessary and unjustified. They can result in civil litigation against the police officers for use of force in wrongful death actions for, even if the situation was a suicide-by-cop, police officers must make reasonable efforts to avoid deadly force. Third, they may result in severe stress for the police officer, and it is this problem that we will discuss in the present chapter.

Vernon Geberth (1993) has noted that police officers who kill the perpetrator in a suicide-by-cop situation often become depressed and angry when they realize that they were used as agents of death for a suicidal perpetrator. The officers may be shattered, devastated by the incident. Officers report feelings of terror during the incident and agitation afterwards. They second-guess their decisions. Should they have fired or waited? Should they have tried to disarm or wound the perpetrator? The officers may suffer flashbacks, experience nightmares and insomnia, and become irritable and hypersensitive. They may lose their self-confidence, which impairs their performance when dealing with possibly armed and dangerous offenders in the future. Will they hesitate to shoot in situations where shooting is required?

Richard Parent and Simon Verdun-Jones (1998) found that three out of 20 (15%) of municipal police officers in British Columbia (Canada) involved in a fatal shooting during the period 1980 to 1995 later quit the force, two as a direct result of the shooting incident. Dean Scoville (1998) reported the case of a police officer, who had killed a suspect in a suicide-by-cop incident, who became morbidly fascinated by such incidents and eventually was involved in another incident in which a man shot himself in the head while this officer was talking to him. This officer committed suicide 18 months later!

If the family of the perpetrator files a civil suit or if the media attacks the police officer and police department because of the incident, this will add to the stress experienced by the police officer.

In some cases, the distress experienced by the police officer may be so strong and prolonged that it amounts to a Post-Traumatic Stress Disorder. Estimates are that this may occur in 5 percent of officers involved in suicide-by-cop incidents. One third may experience moderate or severe reactions, and over 85 percent transitory reactions. Dean Scoville noted that the incident commanders, who have to order police officers to shoot at a perpetrator, may also suffer from post-traumatic stress.

Rivard, Dietz, Martell, and Widawaski (2002) surveyed over a hundred police officers who had been involved in a variety of shooting incidents. They found that 11.3 percent had experienced one or more symptoms of post-traumatic stress disorder (PTSD) and 2.7 percent fulfilled the criteria for a diagnosis of post-traumatic stress disorder. Rivard also studied an acute form of PTSD called acute stress disorder (ASD) which, as it name implies, does not persist for as long as PTSD. Rivard found that 81.3 percent of the police officers experienced one or more symptoms of ASD, and 6.1 percent met the criteria for a diagnosis of ASD. Rivard found that symptoms of ASD were associated with greater levels of depression in the police officers. Although Rivard studied police officers involved in a variety of shooting incidents, the same findings would be expected for those involved in suicide-by-cop incidents.

Typically, the police officers involved are removed from the scene, and the officers may have the weapons they used exchanged for others. They will be interviewed by other police officers, either from a special unit set-up for this purpose or from a regular unit (such as the Homicide Department). They may be removed from active duty and assigned to a desk job.

As a result, police officers involved in suicide-by-cop situations need crisis intervention and, sometimes, long-term counseling. Some police departments have set up peer-support for these officers.

Interestingly, very little research has been conducted on this problem. This is in contrast to an analogous situation, when the driver of a subway train runs over a suicide who jumps in front of his train. Let us look at some of the writing on this topic.

HELPING THE TRAIN DRIVER WHO
RUNS OVER A PASSENGER

In the London (England) subway (known to Londoners as the Tube), Ian O'Donnell and Richard Farmer (1994) calculated that an average of 94 people jumped in front of the trains each year in the 1980s. In the Hong Kong subway, Mark Gaylord and David Lester (1994) counted 50 completed suicides and a further 60 attempted suicides in the 1980s.

T. Tranah and Richard Farmer (1994) interviewed 76 drivers who experienced a person jumping or falling in front of their train. The drivers took an average of 21 sick days after the trauma. Thirteen of the drivers (17%) were diagnosed as having a post-traumatic stress disorder, and a further 12 (16%) were found to have lesser psychiatric problems (primarily depression and phobias). Thus, one-third of the drivers had a serious adverse reaction to the incident. Six months later, however, only two of the drivers were still upset enough to warrant a psychiatric diagnosis.

In Sweden, Theorell, Leymann, Jodko, Kowarski, and Norbeck (1994) followed-up drivers who had run over someone. Compared to drivers who had not experienced such a trauma, the traumatized drivers took more sick days in the first three weeks and, overall, in the first year: 38 percent of the traumatized group but only 14 percent of the comparison group took a month of sick days during months four through 12 of that first year. This excessive absenteeism was greater for drivers for whom the victim was seriously injured or killed than for those involved in incidents in which the victim was only mildly injured. The traumatized drivers had persistent and strong phyisological reactions and increased sleep disturbance, and they described their work situation as getting worse over the year.

D. Tang (1994), in Denmark, described a 22-year-old driver who was driving his train at 60 kilometers an hour and ran over a woman sitting on the tracks. He felt shock, started trembling, and felt nauseous. He was unable to talk to the passengers over the intercom. He did not leave the cabin to inspect the victim, but her husband entered the train later and told the driver that his wife suffered from manic-depressive disorder.

After the investigation, the driver was sent home in a taxi. He opted to visit his girlfriend rather than talk to a counselor. However, he experienced anxiety and depression, was preoccupied with trying to understand the woman's motives, and had fantasies of her mutilated body. He also had trouble speaking, losing his voice on occasions.

The driver seriously considered resigning from his job and finally sought psychotherapy. Tang first set him up with a speech therapist. Then he worked to help the driver overcome his fear of driving in the dark, accompanying him on the train as he drove it. Tang also explained to the driver that the thoughts and fantasies which the driver was having were to be expected and not signs of mental illness.

Tang felt that drivers should be warned about the psychological consequences of traumatic incidents during their training. They should also be told about the usefulness of counseling. Supervisors should be reminded of this from time to time in re-training sessions. After an incident, crisis intervention in the first 24 hours is crucial, with crisis counselors available to go directly to the station where the incident has occurred. This should be followed by long-term therapy if the situation requires it. In Norway, O. Foss (1994) noted that strong support from colleagues was of great help to traumatized drivers.

Williams, Miller, Watson, and Hunt (1994) noted that it is useful if the organization has a standardized debriefing procedure established, followed by year-long follow-up, especially when the driver returns to work, prior to the inquest and at the one-year anniversary of the incident. The debriefing must be supportive and clearly not an investigation. It should be mandatory for all drivers involved in incidents so that no driver feels singled out for attention and no driver feels compelled to be "macho" and decline to attend.

The debriefing meeting should look for signs of distress and adjustment, discuss the effects to be expected, and check issues concerned with job satisfaction and competence. The driver should be reassured on his return to work that all will not go as before with him. He must expect over-vigilance and concentration difficulties, anxiety, and reduced job satisfaction.

We have been impressed by the careful study and thought given to the trauma experienced by train drivers, and we regret that not as much attention has been given to police officers who experience trauma.

HELPING THOSE WITH POST-TRAUMATIC STRESS

For a strict psychiatric diagnosis of post-traumatic stress disorder as defined by the American Psychiatric Association, the patient must suffer from three clusters of symptoms. First, the patient must re-experience the trauma from time to time, with such symptoms as nightmares, flashbacks, and intrusive thoughts. Second, the patient must show avoidance behaviors, with symptoms such as emotional numbing and an inability to recall aspects of the traumatic event. Third, the patient must show arousal, with symptoms such as insomnia and an extreme startle response to stimuli.

Richard Bryant (2000) has described the variety of techniques which can be used to help those with post-traumatic stress. The patient's anxiety level can be reduced by means of systematic desensitization, a process in which the patient is presented with very weak anxiety-arousing stimuli, all the while being helped to relax. Over the course of sessions spread over several weeks, the stimuli presented to the patient get stronger and stronger (that is, more closely similar to the traumatic event itself), until he or she can tolerate the stimuli with minimal anxiety.

Sometimes the patient can be exposed to the feared stimuli either in reality (a process called flooding) or in fantasy (a process called implosive therapy). The patient will feel extreme anxiety, but the physiological response of the patient cannot maintain itself for a long time at a high level, and eventually the patient becomes less physiologically aroused in the presence of the feared stimuli (a process called habituation).

In cognitive therapy, the therapist helps patients examine the thoughts they have, especially those relevant to the traumatic event and its consequences. Often these are irrational, and the therapist points this out and helps the patients change the irrational thoughts to rational thoughts. For example, after not handling an incident well, a person may think, "I always mess up. I am a total incompetent." The therapist may challenge the "always"—the person is unlikely to *always* mess up. The therapist may also challenge the self-labeling, suggesting that the person is not an incompetent, but rather someone who sometimes, but probably not often, does not perform up to his or her abilities.

Finally, Bryant mentioned eye movement desensitization and reprocessing which requires the patient to focus attention on a traumatic memory while visually tracking the therapist's finger as it moves. Bryant noted that this technique is controversial, with some commentators claiming that it has no therapeutic value while others claim that it is beneficial to patients.

CRITICAL INCIDENT DEBRIEFING

It has become common in recent years for crisis interveners and counselors to be available for those who have experienced a traumatic situation. This process is come called "critical incident debriefing."

Everly, Flannery, and Mitchell (2000) have noted that this process should more properly be called critical incident stress management, and it should include pre-crisis procedures as well. Agencies should be prepared for critical incidents and have well-thought-out procedures in place before incidents occur. Furthermore, the training of staff should include segments which prepare the staff for the traumatic events they may encounter.

Once critical incidents occur, there should be opportunities for individuals to have acute crisis counseling, brief small group discussions (defusings) to assist the reduction of acute symptoms, longer small group discussions (called debriefings), family crisis counseling where appropriate (and this may especially important for the families of police officers who themselves may suffer stress from the officer's involvement in a critical incident), referral opportunities for long-term counseling, and follow-up procedures to ensure that the officer continues to improve. In general, those involved in traumatic situations are encouraged to tell their stories, share their responses to the traumatic events, are informed of the typical responses to such events, and helped to gain closure about the experience.

Michael McMains and Wayman Mullins (1996) have suggested that this debriefing is useful, not only for the police officers involved in these situations, but also for the hostages if there were any, and even for the perpetrator. In this latter case, the debriefing maintains rapport with the perpetrator, assures him that he did the right thing by surrendering, and reinforces the fact that you kept your side of all the bargaining and did everything you could to meet his demands. Some perpetrators repeat the offense, and this debriefing helps working with the perpetrator if similar situations arise in the future.

McMains and Mullins note that an "operational" debriefing is useful. What are the facts of the situation and what happened? They suggest developing a standardized review protocol so that all of the available information is collected, including such data as:

the date
local time
place
hostage data
offender data

circumstances
weapons/explosives
measures taken by the police
    initial police action
    command post
    specialty teams involved
    technical equipment and support
    other measures
negotiations
final stages of the incident
persons killed or wounded
legal aspects
review and evaluation

McMains and Mullins suggest that the emotional debriefing should take place in a group setting, with the police officers involved present, along with officers professionally-trained in critical incident debriefing, but with no ranking officers present. The purpose is to review what happened to the people during the incident, how each person felt about what happened, and to provide information about the typical reactions experienced as a result of such traumatic situations.

Many people involved in traumatic incidents experience emotions and have thoughts that they consider to be deviant or pathological in some way. Is it normal to feel anger or anxiety and guilt as a result of your actions? Is it normal to have no emotional response, to feel emotionally numb? The participants in the debriefing need to be reassured by the professionals that all these reactions and non-reactions are common, and the participants will feel relieved to see that others have experienced and are experiencing the same emotions and thoughts.

John Curtis (1995) has described the elements involved in this process in greater detail. First, the counselor may have to help clients recognize the emotions and thoughts which are occurring in their mind. The clients may be experiencing fear, anger, and guilt, but may not recognize the presence of these emotions. Questions such as "Are you feeling helpless?" move clients toward this recognition. However, the counselor should not suggest the presence of these emotions too soon in the counseling process, for clients may not be able to handle these emotions immediately after the trauma. Related to this, the counselor may have to label the emotions for the clients. The clients may be emotionally aroused but not be able to label the emotions accurately. Statements such as "You sound angry" may move clients toward accurate labelling of their emotions. Counselors may have to suggest negative emotions and thoughts to the clients in order to accelerate the de-traumatization process.

The clients must be helped to "get in touch" with their experience. Talking about the experience is useful, but not sufficient. At some point in time, clients must re-experience the emotional states so that these emotions can dissipate. The counselor may have to indicate that it is helpful to ventilate and that responses such as crying, screaming, and swearing are normal and useful in the healing process.

The counselor must indicate to the clients during the debriefing process after the stand-off that their behavior has been courageous and something to be proud of. This validation of the clients' behavior encourages further communication and ventilation, for clients will often re-experience the trauma by themselves many times before the emotional charge of the traumatic experience is fully discharged. Counselors should also help the client accept the traumatic situation by reframing it, for example, as a possible growth experience, so that the clients can see the trauma and debriefing as a constructive event.

As we noted above, some participants in the debriefing may experience more long-lasting effects, even to the extent of suffering from post-traumatic stress disorder. Others may experience anxiety attacks. In these cases, more extensive therapy may be required from psychotherapists using the wide variety of techniques that they have available, ranging from medications, cognitive therapy to behavior therapy.

SUICIDE-BY-COP

In suicide-by-cop situations, the trauma for the police officers may be especially great. The majority of barricade situations are resolved without loss of life—the FBI has estimated that 95 percent end in this satisfactory way. Thus, the death of the perpetrator (and perhaps of hostages, if there were any) is unusual, thereby increasing the sense of failure on the part of the police officers.

Furthermore, the police officer or officers who actually killed the perpetrator may find out that the man did not have a lethal weapon, even though he appeared to have one. For example, the gun he was pointing toward the police officers may have been unloaded. The perpetrator may have planned to force the police officers to kill him as a means of committing suicide.

As a result, the police officers responsible for the death of the perpetrator may feel anger and guilt over their actions, as well as anxiety over how their superiors and the media will react to the events.

In one video shown at the FBI Academy during a conference on suicide-by-cop, such a police officer is seen standing by himself at the side of a roadway while others deal with the crime scene. He is obviously tense, and no one is there with him to offer support.

Police officers involved in suicide-by-cop incidents may also suffer a loss of status in the police department. They may be assigned to the "rubber gun" department, that is, have their gun taken away from them and assigned to desk duty. There is also stigma among police officers in visiting a therapist or a "shrink." Thus, police officers may undergo additional stress after the incident which, for example, the train drivers in the examples given earlier do not experience.

It is clear, therefore, that helping the police officer involved in a suicide-by-cop incident is of crucial importance. Police departments should set up sound procedures to accomplish this task as part of their Employee Assistance Program. There should be critical incident debriefing, peer support programs, and the availability of individual counseling with a psychologist.

CRITICISMS OF PSYCHOLOGICAL DEBRIEFING

There is a growing number of critics who argue that psychological debriefing, critical incident debriefing, and post-trauma counseling is of little use, can sometimes result in harm, and has dangerous social and political implications. The mental health professionals involved have been called "modern ambulance chasers" who "create victims" (Anon, 2003). Vanessa Pupavac (2001), for example, views PTSD as a label given to whole populations who experience an event and who are experiencing the *normal* coping responses. In her view, PTSD is the "disorder du jour" which became popular in mental health circles because of lobbying by veterans of the Vietnam War and their supporters. It is based on the notion that individuals are universally vulnerable, and that resilience and coping are seen as "denial" and, therefore, evidence of psychological dysfunction. Pupavac suggests that those who are attracted to counseling as a profession are often those who are former patients and that they are projecting their own sense of psychological vulnerability onto others. At the social level, psychological debriefing can be seen as a tactic by the professional and managerial classes to define what is normal behavior and to impose non-punitive psychiatric sanctions on those who are deviant. It is a way of imposing social control.

These are strong words! Is there any evidence to back up this position? Jonathan Bisson and Martin Deahl (1994) noted that sound research on this issue is lacking because many of the studies have methodological flaws. However, it is possible to find research that finds no beneficial impact from psychological debriefing. For example, in a study of soldiers who handled and identified the dead during the Gulf War, those who received psychological debriefing and those who did not had a similar incidence of psychiatric problems nine months later (Deahl, Gillham, Thomas, Searle, and Srinivasan, 1994). A study of burn patients assigned randomly to groups receiving psychological interventions and those receiving none found that the two groups did not differ 13 months later at follow-up in reduced functioning, occupational change, or increased alcohol intake or smoking. Those receiving psychological interventions scored worse on measures of anxiety and depression at follow-up and worse on a measure of the impact of the trauma.

Much more research is needed on this issue, an issue on which those advocating either position feel very strongly about. At the present time, all we can do is learn the techniques used in psychological debriefing and remain aware that there is the possibility that such interventions may not be effective and may, perhaps, cause harm to some clients.

CHAPTER 14

How to Lessen the Incidence of Suicide-by-Cop

How can we prevent suicide-by-cop? First, we must develop more information on incidents of suicide-by-cop so that we can develop a profile of the typical suicide-by-cop incident. If we could collect several hundred incidents from around the country and code them for perpetrator characteristics and the circumstances of the situation, we would then have a sense of the "typical" suicide-by-cop incident.

However, not all suicide-by-cop incidents are the same, and so the second step is to identify types of suicide-by-cop incidents, both for perpetrators and for situations. If these types are found to be reliable, then we can take the circumstances of a specific suicide-by-cop incident and determine what kind of perpetrator we have, how the incident will probably develop, and what techniques have been found to work with this particular type of suicide-by-cop incident. For this, it is crucial that mental health professionals, researchers, and police departments cooperate, for each of these groups can contribute specialized skills to the investigations.

Interestingly, however, Robert Homant and his colleagues (2000) reviewed 123 incidents of suicide-by-cop from a variety of sources and concluded "There do not seem to be any obvious training implications here . . ." (p. 50). They did recommend that the perpetrators should be treated as dangerous, that police should not force the perpetrator's hand, and that the perpetrator should be safely contained.

Homant's conclusion is unduly negative. Information is of great use in planning the response to suicide-by-cop incidents. It is especially important to review each suicide-by-cop incident afterwards to document what tactics were used and to compare the results of the tactics with the characteristics of the incident and the perpetrator.

In this way, information can be developed on which tactics work best in each type of incident and with each kind of perpetrator.

Then, once we have developed reliable information on suicide-by-cop incidents, this information, along with its implications for police responses, must be incorporated into the initial training of police officers and provided in refresher courses from time to time. This will help police officers identify and respond to a suicide-by-cop situation.

DEFUSING

In an Associated Press report in June 1998, Kevin Gilmartin, a former hostage negotiator, was quoted as saying the police departments frequently rely too heavily on SWAT teams, high-tech weapons, and "surgical" shooting techniques. A skilled negotiator can often defuse a situation without any injury or death to the participants. If a stand-off with a civilian can be diagnosed as a suicide-by-cop situation, and if the situation does not escalate too quickly, then non-lethal, or less lethal, tactics can be employed.

Tactical withdrawal can lessen the speed with which a suicide-by-cop incident escalates. The more physical distance between the perpetrator and the police, the less likely the police will be threatened, and the police officers will be less likely to use deadly force. The result is more time for the police to formulate a plan of action. Withdrawal may also calm the perpetrator and neutralize his actions and suicidal intentions. Dean Scoville (1998) suggested that a suicidal perpetrator, in an area by himself and where no one else is at risk, can be left alone. The longer a confrontation is delayed by the police officers, the better.

Subjects visibly wielding weapons other than firearms or bombs can be dealt with using less-than-lethal force. A knife-wielding perpetrator, for example, who is more than 21 feet away from police officers, can sometimes be disarmed using shotgun-projected bean bags or rubber bullets. In these cases, Dean Scoville recommended that a designated sharp-shooter have the perpetrator in his sights should the perpetrator quickly close the distance between himself and the police officers.

These approaches are appropriate, of course, if the perpetrator is alone. If the perpetrator has hostages and is threatening their lives, defusing tactics like these cannot be employed. Saving the lives of the hostages becomes a greater priority than saving the life of the perpetrator.

The above comments apply to situations in which the suicide-by-cop situation is prolonged, for then there is time to find out about the perpetrator and to plan tactics. However, some situations take place in a brief period of time. Richard Parent (1998a) presented one case which took 21 seconds.

Police officers were called to a residence where it was reported that a man had stabbed himself and was "freaking people out." Two officers arrived and approached the residence. A man left the residence brandishing a butcher's knife. He approached the officers who separated from each other in the yard and drew their firearms. The man was ordered to drop the knife, whereupon he told the police officers to shoot him. He then advanced toward one of the officers. He was again told to drop the knife, but he continued to advance. When he was six feet from the officer, both officers fired, killing him. One of the officers said:

> It all happened so fast. I fired as soon as I could. He wanted to die. He said shoot me. He was crazed; he had that thousand-yard stare . . . that nothing look behind his eyes. It wasn't a stand-off; he was gonna kill me. I could have run, but I would have had to turn and I would have got stabbed. (Parent, 1998a, p. 8)

Interestingly, the coroner's jury ruled the death to be a suicide.

THE USE OF NON-LETHAL WEAPONS

One suggestion for lessening the incidence of suicide-by-cop is to equip police officers with more kinds of nonlethal weapons, such as pepper spray, net guns, glue guns, Taser guns (which discharge electric probes), and grappling poles and shields. These weapons are not always widely available to police officers. Often then are given only to special units. They are quite expensive and require additional training in their use.

It has been documented in earlier chapters that, on occasions, the perpetrator of a suicide-by-cop incident does not always have a loaded or operational firearm. In these cases, the killing of the perpetrator by police officers may seem unnecessary. However, the majority of suicide-by-cop perpetrators do have functional firearms, and some law enforcement experts caution against using less-than-lethal weapons to eliminate the danger posed by the perpetrator. Dean Scoville gave an example of an elderly man in Southern California who was wielding a revolver. When the police officers fired shotgun-projected bean bags at him to try to disarm him, he fired several shots, wounding one of the police officers. Scoville also noted that the perpetrator may have booby-trapped his person or property, and this may result in police officers who use less-than-lethal weapons being seriously injured or killed.

COMMENT

It is clear that much more investigation of suicide-by-cop is required before we can put forward adequate proposals for preventing injuries and deaths when police officers try to end these incidents. However, the phenomenon of suicide-by-cop has been recognized for only 10 years or so, and so it is too soon to be discouraged in our efforts. We are sure that the next 10 years will see a great advance in our understanding of this phenomenon and much better suggestions for responding to the incidents.

References

Anon. (2003). Mind how you go. *The Economist, 366*(8314), 55.

Andriolo, K. R. (1998). Gender and the cultural construction of good and bad suicides. *Suicide & Life-Threatening Behavior, 28,* 37-49.

Arboleda-Florez, J. (1979). Amok. *Bulletin of the American Academy of Psychiatry & the Law, 7,* 286-295.

Associated Press. (1998, June 8). "Suicide by cop" makes victims of both sides. *Lubbock Avalanche-Journal,* 1-9.

Baechler, J. (1979). *Suicides.* New York: Basic Books.

Berman, A. (1979). Dyadic death. *Suicide & Life-Threatening Behavior, 9,* 15-23.

Bisson, J. I., & Deahl, M. P. (1994). Psychological debriefing and prevention of post-traumatic stress. *British Journal of Psychiatry, 165,* 717-720.

Bisson, J. I., Jenkins, P. L., Alexander, J., & Bannister, C. (1997). Randomised controlled trial of psychological debriefing for victims of acute burn trauma. *British Journal of Psychiatry, 171,* 78-81.

Bohm, R. M. (1999). *Deathquest.* Cincinnati: Anderson.

Boyette, M., & Boyette, R. (1989). *Let it burn!* Chicago: Contemporary Books.

Bresler, S., Scalora, M. J., Elbogen, E. B., & Moore, Y. S. (2003). Attempted suicide by cop. *Journal of Forensic Sciences, 48,* 190-194.

Bryant, R. A. (2000). Cognitive-behavioral therapy of violence-related post-traumatic stress disorder. *Aggression & Violent Behavior, 5,* 79-97.

Burton-Bradley, B. G. (1968). The amok syndrome in Papua and New Guinea. *Medical Journal of Australia, i,* 252-256.

Cialdini, R. B. (1984). *Influence.* New York: William Morrow.

Constantelos, D. J. (1978). The "neomartyrs" as evidence for methods and motives leading to conversion and martyrdom in the Ottoman Empire. *Greek Orthodox Theological Review, 23,* 216-234.

Curtis, J. M. (1995). Elements of critical incident debriefing. *Psychological Reports, 77,* 91-96.

Deahl, M. P., Gillham, A. B., Thomas, J., Searle, M. M., & Srinivasan, M. (1994). Psychological sequelae following the Gulf War. *British Journal of Psychiatry, 165,* 60-65.

Donner, F. (1990). *Protectors of privilege.* Berkeley, CA: University of California.

Dorpat, T. L. (1966, June 27). Suicide in murderers. *Psychiatric Digest,* 51-55.

Dorpat, T. L. (1968). Psychiatric observations on assassinations. *Northwest Medicine, 67,* 976-979.

Eells, G. (1991). *Final Gig.* San Diego: Harcourt Brace Jovanovich.

Everly, G. S., Flannery, R. B., & Mitchell, J. T. (2000). Critical incident stress management (CISM). *Aggression & Violent Behavior, 5,* 23-40.

Fabing, H. D. (1956). On going berserk. *American Journal of Psychiatry, 113,* 409-415.

Foote, W. E. (1999). Victim-precipitated homicide. In H. V. Hall (Ed.) *Lethal violence* (pp. 175-202). Boca Raton, FL: CRC Press.

Foss, O. T. (1994). Mental first aid. *Social Science & Medicine, 38,* 479-482.

Fuselier, G. D., Van Zandt, C. R., & Lancely, F. J. (1989). Negotiating the protracted incident. *FBI Law Enforcement Bulletin, 58*(7), 1-7.

Fuselier, G. D., Van Zandt, C. R., & Lancely, F. J. (1991). Hostage/barricade incidents. *FBI Law Enforcement Bulletin, 60*(1), 6-12.

Gaylord, M. S., & Lester, D. (1994). Suicide in the Hong Kong subway. *Social Science & Medicine, 38,* 427-430.

Geberth, V. (1993, July 7). Suicide-by-cop. *Law & Order, 41,* 105-109.

Geberth, V. J. (1994, January 1). The racial component in suicide-by-cop incidents. *Law & Order, 42,* 318-319.

Geller, W. A., & Scott, M. S. (1992). *Deadly force: What we know.* Washington, DC: Police Executive Research Forum.

Gibbs, J. T. (1988). Conceptual, methodological, and sociocultural issues in Black youth suicide. *Suicide & Life-Threatening Behavior, 18,* 73-89.

Gilmore, M. (1994). *Shot in the heart.* New York: Doubleday.

Hanzlick, R., & Goodin, J. (1997). Mind your manners. *American Journal of Forensic Medicine & Pathology, 18,* 228-245.

Harding, R., & Fahey, R. (1973). Killings by Chicago police, 1969-1970. *Southern California Law Review, 46,* 284-315.

Harner, M. (1972). *The Jivaro.* Garden City, NY: Doubleday.

Harruff, R. C., Llewellyn, A. L., Clark, M. A., Hawley, D. A., & Pless, J. E. (1994). Firearm suicides during confrontations with police. *Journal of Forensic Sciences, 39,* 402-411.

Homant, R. J., & Kennedy, D. B. (2000a). Suicide by police. *Policing, 23,* 339-355.

Homant, R. J., & Kennedy, D. B. (2000b). Effectiveness of less than lethal force in suicide-by-cop incidents. *Police Quarterly, 3,* 153-171.

Homant, R. J., Kennedy, D. B., & Hupp, R. T. (2000). Real and perceived danger in police officer assisted suicide. *Journal of Criminal Justice, 28,* 43-52.

Howze, B. (1977). Suicide. *Journal of Non-White Concerns, 5,* 65-72.

Hughes, R. (1986). *The fatal shore.* New York: Vintage Books.

Hutson, H. R., Anglin, D., Yarbrough, J., Hardaway, K., Russell, M., Strote, J., Canter, M., & Blum, B. (1998). Suicide by cop. *Annals of Emergency Medicine, 32,* 665-669.

Jenet, R. N., & Segal, R. J. (1985). Provoked shooting by police as a mechanism for suicide. *American Journal of Forensic Medicine & Pathology, 6,* 274-275.

Kennedy, D. B., Homant, R. J., & Hupp, R. T. (1998). Suicide by cop. *FBI Law Enforcement Bulletin, 67*(8), 21-27.

Kiev, A. (1972). *Transcultural psychiatry.* New York: Free Press.

Klinger, D. A. (2001). Suicidal intent in victim-precipitated homicide. *Homicide Studies, 5,* 206-226.

Kobler, A. (1975). Figures (and perhaps some facts) on police killings of civilians in the US 1965-1969. *Journal of Social Issues, 31*(1), 185-191.

Lavergne, G. M. (1997). *A sniper in the tower.* Denton, TX: University of North Texas.

Lester, D. (1987). Murder followed by suicide in those who murder police officers. *Psychological Reports, 60,* 1130.

Lester, D. (1988). Suicide and life insurance. *Psychological Reports, 63,* 920.

Lester, D. (1998a). *Suicide in African Americans.* Commack, NY: Nova Science.

Lester, D. (1998b). *The death penalty.* Springfield, IL: Charles Thomas.

Lester, D., & Lester, G. (1975). *Crime of passion.* Chicago: Nelson-Hall.

Lord, V. B. (1999). *One form of victim-precipitated homicide.* Paper presented at the FBI Academy conference on Police Suicide, Quantico, Virginia.

Lord, V. B. (2000). Law-enforcement assisted suicide. *Criminal Justice & Behavior, 27,* 401-419.

Lowie, R. H. (1913). Military societies of the Crow Indians. *Anthropological Papers of the American Museum of Natural History, 11*(3), 143-227.

MacDonald, J. M. (1961). *The murderer and his victim.* Springfield, IL: Charles Thomas.

McMains, M. J., & Mullins, W. C. (1996). *Crisis negotiations.* Cincinnati, OH: Anderson.

Menninger, K. (1938). *Man against himself.* New York: Harcourt, Brace & World.

Miller, R. D. (2001). Suicide by cop and criminal responsibility. *Journal of Psychiatry & Law, 29,* 295-328.

Mohandie, K., & Meloy, J. R. (2000). Clinical and forensic indicators of "suicide by cop." *Journal of Forensic Sciences, 45,* 384-389.

Noesner, G. W., & Dolan, J. T. (1992). First responder training. *FBI Law Enforcement Bulletin, 61*(8), 1-4.

O'Donnell, I., & Farmer, R. D. T. (1994). The epidemiology of suicide on the London Underground. *Social Science & Medicine, 38,* 409-418.

Parent, R. (1998). Invitation to death! *Canadian Security, 20*(1), 22-23.

Parent, R. B. (1998). Victim-precipitated homicide. *Royal Canadian Mounted Police Gazette, 60*(4), 2-14.

Parent, R. B., & Verdun-Jones, S. (1998). Victim-precipitated homicide. *Policing, 21,* 432-448.

Parker, S. (1960). The Wiitiko psychosis in the context of Ojibwa personality and culture. *American Anthropologist, 62,* 603-623.

Pearson, H. (1994). *The shadow of the Panthers.* Reading, MA: Addison-Wesley.

Pupavac, V. (2001, April 10-12). *The end of politics?* Paper presented at the 51st Political Studies Association Conference, Manchester, United Kingdom.

Rivard, J. M., Dietz, P., Martell, D., & Widawaski, M. (2002). Acute dissociative responses in law enforcement officers involved in critical shooting incidents. *Journal of Forensic Sciences, 47,* 1093-1100.

Robin, G. (1963). Justifiable homicide by police officers. *Journal of Criminal Law, Criminology & Police Science, 54,* 225-231.

Scolville, D. (1998, November). Getting you to pull the trigger. *Police,* 36-44.

Sellin, T. (1959). *The death penalty.* Philadelphia: American Law Institute.

Sophocles. (1956). *The Theban plays.* Translated by E. F. Watling. Baltimore: Penguin.

Stincelli, R. Suicide-by-cop. http://iiiconfess.com/SBC.html

Stone, I. F. (1988). *The trial of Socrates.* Boston: Little Brown.

Tang, D. (1994). Psychotherapy for train drivers after railway suicide. *Social Science & Medicine, 38,* 477-478.

Theorell, T., Leymann, H., Jodko, M., Kowarski, K., & Norbeck, H. E. (1994). "Person under train" incidents from the subway driver's point of view. *Social Science & Medicine, 38,* 471-475.

Tranah, T., & Farmer, R. D. T. (1994). Psychological reactions of drivers to railway suicide. *Social Science & Medicine, 38,* 459-469.

Ury, W. (1991). *Getting past No.* New York: Bantam.

Valentine, C. A., & Valentine, B. L. (1972). The man and the Panthers. *Politics & Society, 2,* 273-286.

van Wormer, K. (1995). Execution-inspired murder: A form of suicide? *Journal of Offender Rehabilitation, 22*(3/4), 1-10.

Van Wulfften-Palthe, P. M. (1936). Psychiatry and neurology in the tropics. In C. D. de Langan & A. Lichtenstein (Eds.), *A clinical textbook of tropical medicine* (pp. 525-547). Batavia, NY: Kolff.

Van Zandt, C. R. (n.d.). *Suicide by cop.* Unpublished paper.

Wertham, F. (1949). *The show of violence.* Garden City, NY: Doubleday.

West, D. J. (1966). *Murder followed by suicide.* Cambridge, MA: Harvard University Press.

Westermeyer, J. (1972). A comparison of amok and other homicide in Laos. *American Journal of Psychiatry, 129,* 703-709.

Westermeyer, J. (1973). Grenade-amok in Laos. *International Journal of Social Psychiatry, 19,* 251-260.

Williams, C., Miller, J., Watson, G., & Hunt, N. (1994). A strategy for trauma debriefing after railway suicides. *Social Science & Medicine, 38,* 483-487.

Wilson, E. F., Davis, J. H., Bloom, J. D., Batten, P. J., & Kamara, S. G. (1998). Homicide or suicide? *Journal of Forensic Sciences, 43,* 46-52.

Wolfgang, M. E. (1958). *Patterns of criminal homicide.* Philadelphia: University of Pennsylvania.

Wolfgang, M. E. (1959). Suicide by means of victim-precipitated homicide. *Journal of Clinical & Experimental Psychopathology, 20,* 335-349.

Index

For Product Safety Concerns and Information please contact our EU
representative GPSR@taylorandfrancis.com Taylor & Francis Verlag GmbH,
Kaufingerstraße 24, 80331 München, Germany

Printed and bound by CPI Group (UK) Ltd, Croydon, CR0 4YY
01/05/2025
01859201-0001